Yoga for the Special Child

A Therapeutic Approach for Infants and Children with Down Syndrome, Cerebral Palsy, and Learning Disabilities

Sonia Sumar

Special Yoga Publications
Buckingham, Virginia

Printed in the United States of America

Special Yoga Publications
Route 1, Box 1559
Buckingham, VA 23921
Tel: (804) 969-2668
Fax: (804) 969-1962
Email: Info@specialyoga.com
Web: www.specialyoga.com

Text and cover design by Bookwrights Press

ISBN: 0-9658024-0-X

Library of Congress Catalogue Card Number: 97-91925

Note: The techniques, ideas, and teaching methods in this book are not intended as a substitute for professional medical advice. Consult your child's pediatrician or specialist before beginning this or any new exercise routine with your child. Any application of the techniques, ideas, and teaching methods in this book is at the reader's sole discretion and risk.

Dedication

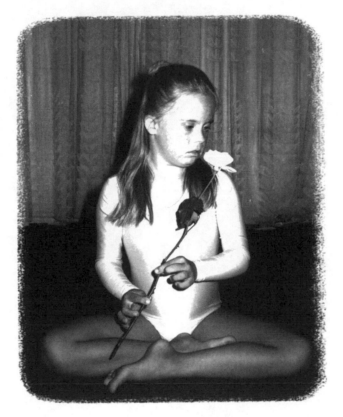

In loving memory of my daughter Roberta

Contents

Foreword

To the Original Portuguese Edition

We all know how good yoga is for the physical body and for the mind, providing health, beauty, mental control, and emotional stability. It was through yoga that Sonia Sumar was able to achieve the incredible results she presents in this book. A real song of hope!

In a simple and clear style, Sonia offers her message of transformation and love. This book is a true treasure that speaks to the heart and helps make the world a better place.

Among yoga colleagues, Sonia is acknowledged as an authority due to her work with children who have special needs. Now she offers us the amazing results in case histories of her daughter and other special yoga students. This is just a part of the lovely, noble, and great mission that Sonia is carrying out. She has become a model for the mothers of these children! Her sincere words convey a sublime message, teaching us how to accept reality joyfully and how to achieve and maintain our inner peace.

If Sonia's suggestions are followed at home, the health and happiness of the entire family will improve. Her work is an example of preventive medicine and solidarity with our brothers and sisters. It is just like the sun—shedding light, warmth, and blessing.

My sincere honor and admiration.

Prof. Maria da Glória Moreira de Souza
Belo Horizonte, Brazil

Introduction

I began to practice yoga during my last year of college in Nilopolis, near my home town of Nova Iguaçu, in the state of Rio de Janeiro, Brazil. My goal was not just better health. On a deeper level, I was hoping to realize some of the mental and psychological benefits that I had read about in a book on yoga. These benefits include mindfulness, concentration, emotional balance, and, ultimately, peace of mind and happiness. The results of my yoga practice were soon forthcoming: I began to experience a heightened degree of mental clarity and a new sense of physical and emotional well-being.

In February 1972 the birth of my second daughter, Roberta, prompted me to enroll in a yoga school and begin a course of practical instruction that would last for several years. Roberta was born with Down Syndrome, a genetic disorder characterized by below-average intelligence and certain physical anomalies. I then began to practice yoga not just for myself, but primarily for Roberta, searching for a key that would unlock the door to a condition considered incurable by medical science.

My work with Roberta began in a way quite natural for the two of us. It was partly experimental and partly intuitive. I did not deviate from traditional yoga teachings, but utilized and adapted those practices and postures that suited Roberta's particular needs. As our rapport and mutual understanding grew, I began to see improvements in her motor coordination, physical strength, and intelligence. Inspired by my success with Roberta, I continued to work with her daily. Her personality and character were developing in a way that was nothing short of amazing. Seeing the new direction my life was taking, I decided to attend training courses to become a yoga teacher.

Several years later, I began to teach yoga at a special education school in Belo Horizonte and became acquainted with many of the parents and teachers there. Even before I opened my own yoga school in January of 1980, I was already receiving telephone calls and letters from many parents of children with disabilities. Disheartened by the lack of support from doctors and other health care professionals, these parents turned to me as their only hope for an alternative, non-surgical approach to their children's problems. Since I had already experienced many of these difficulties myself, I was now in a position to help others. I decided to open my own yoga school.

For the past seventeen years I have continued to operate my yoga school in Belo Horizonte, often traveling to other states in Brazil and abroad for workshops and conferences. In 1983 Ground Press of Brazil published the first edition of *Yoga for the Special Child*; a second edition was published in 1985, and a third in 1994. My purpose in writing this book was to share my experience as a mother and to chronicle the story of my daughter's life, as well as to provide the history and methods of my therapeutic work with other children who have special needs.

In this new English edition of *Yoga for the Special Child*, the text has been expanded to include additional case histories, more detailed instructions for the yoga practitioner, and a greater number of photographs. To accommodate this added material, the book has been divided into two parts. The first part contains a detailed account of Roberta's life, followed by case histories of my students with special needs. The second part is a "hands-on" instruction manual for parents, educators, yoga teachers, and health care professionals. The instruction manual illustrates the yoga techniques and methods that have proven most effective in promoting the development of children with special needs.

At our yoga center, we begin working with each child on an individual basis. In general, the younger the child, the greater the restorative effects of yoga. When the student reaches a certain level of development, he or she is encouraged to join a children's group class. As progress continues, the student may enter an adult class. The majority of my students with disabilities have Down Syndrome; however, I have also used yoga as a therapy for children with cerebral palsy, microcephaly, Prader Willi Syndrome, Cat's Cry Syndrome, learning disabilities, and attention deficit disorder.

Our style of yoga is extremely gentle and safe. It requires no special equipment other than a thick towel or blanket to cushion the floor. Parents, teachers, and other professionals can employ these methods at home, school, or in private therapy sessions.

All our remedial yoga classes follow the same basic outline. The teacher chooses one of several different yoga routines, depending on the age of the child and the degree of motor impairment. Each routine corresponds to a particular stage in the child's development. A typical class for an infant begins with the practice of repetitive movements and physical postures, and ends with a session of guided relaxation. As the child progresses, breathing exercises, sound therapy, and more advanced postures are added to the routine.

At our yoga center we mainstream all our students with special needs into integrated group classes. These classes include children at many different levels of development, both with and without disabilities. Our teaching method is noncompetitive: we encourage each child to perform his or her personal best, with the emphasis on harmony and cooperation. This approach provides a foundation for building mutual trust and self-confidence—important qualities for the success of our program.

During my twenty-three years as a yoga teacher of children with special needs, I have seen many so-called "hopeless cases" respond to the stimulus of a properly designed remedial yoga program. However, there first needs to be a strong conviction on the parents' part that their child has the potential to improve. Sometimes this may seem difficult, especially in the face of opposition and prejudice, but it is an essential ingredient to the success of the program.

By letting go of our fears and negativity, and learning to see the best in ourselves and others, we can provide a powerful impetus for positive change. It is through this ability to go beyond preconceived notions and external appearances that we can transform our lives and those of our children. May all the parents of children with special needs develop this ability, and may they and their children experience true peace and happiness.

Sonia Sumar
Belo Horizonte, Brazil
December 1996

Part One

Narratives

1

The Story of Roberta

How it all Began

My first child, Renata, a healthy girl, was born by Caesarean section on February 3, 1970. When I became pregnant again a year later, I imagined the only difference this time might be the birth of a son or an easier delivery. I had no way to predict the arrival of Roberta, the special child who would alter the entire course of my life, including my career.

Roberta was born on February 26, 1972, in Belo Horizonte, a city of three million, situated some 300 miles north of Rio de Janeiro—the picturesque, old port-city that used to be the capital of Brazil. I had grown up near Rio and met my husband there. Due to a change in my husband's employment in early 1971, our family relocated to Belo Horizonte. Shortly thereafter, I became pregnant with Roberta.

Roberta came into the world by Caesarean section after an extremely long and difficult labor. Because the incision from my first Caesarean had never healed properly, unanticipated delays and complications occurred during this second delivery. By the time Roberta was finally born, she had become cyanosed (a bluish discoloration of the skin resulting from inadequate oxygenation of the blood), and her lungs had filled with amniotic fluid aspirated during delivery. For this reason, she was placed in an incubator, where she spent the next three days receiving oxygen.

For more than fourteen hours after Roberta's birth, I remained in a coma caused by a post-delivery hemorrhage. I finally regained consciousness after receiving a blood transfusion, the first of four during my one-week hospital stay. Very concerned by my loss of blood, my doctor told me it was unlikely I would be able to nurse

Roberta in my weakened state. Up to this point, no milk had formed in my breasts.

I knew how much Roberta had already suffered and wanted to nurse her as soon as possible. I firmly believed it was her biological birthright. Also, because of my experience in nursing Renata, I was aware of the deep bond between mother and child which develops during breast-feeding. I prayed for the return of my physical strength and then waited patiently for nature to take its course in providing the proper nourishment for my child. When the time came for Roberta to be released from the incubator, I was ready to give my daughter her first taste of mother's milk. At first Roberta nursed sparingly. Soon I had so much milk I was able to donate some to another child in the hospital.

The first time I held Roberta, I noticed that her reflexes were considerably slower than what I would have expected. Because it had been such a difficult delivery, the attending pediatrician was hesitant to make a definite diagnosis. He said it was most likely that Roberta had Down Syndrome, but only time would tell.

It goes without saying that no parent wants to give birth to a child with a disability. I certainly never expected to have a baby with Down Syndrome. On the other hand, I never regretted Roberta's birth, nor did I ever feel she was a burden to me. What others might have regarded as a misfortune was for me both a challenge and an opportunity. I did not have to reason out why I felt this way about my daughter. I just knew, and what I knew was something so simple, yet so profound, it dispelled all my doubts: I loved Roberta with all my heart and was firmly resolved to do whatever I could to ensure her future success and happiness.

At first I didn't know how or where to start. I knew very little about Down Syndrome and was unable to pay for a specialist. I also had other responsibilities at home as a mother and housewife. Then I realized I had already begun my work with Roberta— by giving her my milk, my caresses, and my attention, by wanting the best for her, and, above all, by giving her my unconditional love and accepting her just the way she was—Down Syndrome and all.

The First Year

One week after Roberta's birth, we returned home to my husband and two-year-old Renata. I resumed my daily housework, meal preparation, and care of Renata. But now I also had Roberta, and the desire to give her all the attention and affection I felt were so crucial to her development. Every activity with Roberta became an opportunity for me to demonstrate my love for her. When she nursed, I visualized my milk flowing into her little body and filling it with all the nutrition she needed to grow up strong and healthy. When I changed her diaper or gave her a bath, I caressed her tenderly and sang or talked to her lovingly and reassuringly. And when a free moment arrived, I covered her face and body with my kisses.

Several weeks later, the diagnosis of Down Syndrome was confirmed by my pediatrician. Roberta had many of the classical features, including a shortened bone structure, large spaces between the first and second toes, a flattened midface, slightly slanted eyes with epicanthal folds of skin at the inner corners, and a tongue that often extended from her mouth. The structure of her face gave her the appearance of an Oriental, which accounts for the derivation of the term "mongoloid," no longer commonly used because of its racial implications.

In the area of motor activity, her reflexes were unusually slow. When I held her, her body sometimes felt as though it had no bones or form; this characteristic, sometimes referred to as "floppy baby syndrome," is caused by a lack of muscle tone. She was also extremely passive and easy-going most of the time. All of these symptoms, along with Down Syndrome's ever-present mental retardation, arise from a chromosome abnormality present at the time of conception.

I had never read anything about yoga with regard to a disability, nor was I familiar with its use as an infant therapy. Nevertheless, it seemed to me that a system of self-cultivation that developed mental concentration, physical strength, flexibility, and motor coordination, and at the same time was gentle enough for a person of any age to practice, could bring only good results to my daughter. From my own personal experience with yoga, I already knew how safe and effective its methods were in restoring and maintaining physical health and mental function. And my experience was not just an isolated case. Over the centuries, millions of people have practiced yoga and experienced its benefits. Indisputably, yoga has withstood the test of time.

When Roberta reached her third month, I decided to prepare her for the practice of yoga by introducing some of its basic physical postures. These postures, called *asanas*, are properly performed without strain and held only so long as they feel steady and comfortable. At this time Roberta could not even lift her head; I would have to help her practice asanas by guiding her body through the movements of each pose. I decided to begin with an inverted pose. By reversing the pull of gravity, the inverted postures are particularly beneficial to the endocrine glands, as well as to the brain and central nervous system.

I placed Roberta on my bed and turned her over onto her back. Then I grasped her ankles and slowly raised her body into the air until she was completely upside down. At first I was very cautious and held her up for only about fifteen to twenty seconds. After a week or so I began to gradually increase the duration of the posture until I was holding her up for several minutes at a time. Since Roberta did not experience any adverse effects, I continued with this posture daily.

During her fourth month, while Roberta continued to nurse regularly, I introduced fresh fruit juices and purees into her diet. She soon became constipated. In order to stimulate peristalsis in her large intestine, I tried massaging her lower abdomen several times a day. Gradually, her constipation cleared up, and I was able to add other foods to her regimen, including vegetable soups and cereal grains.

Then I began a series of tests and experiments with Roberta in order to evaluate her abilities and help her develop the capacity to respond to different kinds of sensory stimuli. I used colored objects, body movements, and special sounds with changing rhythms. Every day I devised new exercises. It was a trial-and-error method, always with the goal of improving Roberta's concentration, muscle tone, and motor coordination, and at the same time helping her to prepare for the practice of yoga. Creating and executing these exercises was a real challenge for me. As Roberta and I played and learned together, I felt myself becoming more and more attuned to her innermost thoughts and feelings.

At this point I began to realize that Roberta was, in fact, teaching me. My job was to be open and receptive to what her body was trying to tell me and to follow the path of her development, moment to moment and day by day. Even today, I credit Roberta as the true leader in my work with children who have special needs.

In Roberta's sixth month I intensified her training in the area of muscle strengthening exercises. Because she still could not sit up, I decided to concentrate on the lower back and pelvic areas. Placing her in a seated position on my bed with her legs apart, I allowed her body to bend forward until her forehead touched the bed. After about five minutes Roberta began to show signs of discomfort, so I removed her from this position. On the second day she was able to raise her head in the forward-bending position. I placed her hands on the bed, beneath her shoulders, so she could push her body up to a seated position.

During the exercises I always talked to her in a loving and supportive tone of voice. I explained the purpose of our training, my deep belief in her potential for positive change, and the need for her cooperation in our work. Sometimes she seemed to respond; at other times she remained inert, ignoring me completely. After each exercise session I massaged her legs and lower back to help her relax and to stimulate the flow of blood into these areas. At the end of one week, Roberta had already begun to raise her trunk off the bed with the help of her hands.

By her eighth month Roberta could sit on her own and was beginning to crawl. Her concentration span was increasing, and she was starting to pay attention to what was happening around her. I sensed that this would be a good time to expand her practice of yoga by introducing the special yogic breathing exercises called *pranayama*. Pranayama means control of the breath. Its practice helps to increase oxygenation of the blood and to remove toxins from the bloodstream, aiding in the recovery from illness. Among its many benefits, pranayama is a powerful restorative for the central nervous system.

I began with two breathing exercises, the "Bellows Breath" and the "Cleansing Breath." These are noisy and somewhat forced breathing techniques that are easy to follow. Seated next to her on the floor, I would practice on my own, allowing her to observe me without calling attention to what I was doing. At first, Roberta just watched me, amused by the "funny" sounds and diaphragmatic movements. Several days later she began to imitate my actions, and very soon we were practicing pranayama together.

I then added two asanas to Roberta's daily exercise routine: the "Cobra Pose" and the "Bow Pose." Both of these are backward-bending poses that help to develop strength in the back muscles and flexibility in the spine. These poses also exert a beneficial effect on the kidneys and nervous system. A short time later I introduced two forward-bending asanas, one with the legs together and the other with the legs apart.

During her eighth month I weaned Roberta. By this time she already enjoyed a balanced diet that included whole fruits and vegetables, grains, beans, egg yolks, and dairy products in the form of whole milk and yogurt. In addition, she received the benefits of daily sunbaths when possible (avoiding the hours of intense sunlight between 11:00 a.m. and 3:00 p.m.). Though still slightly pudgy, Roberta looked healthy for a child of her age. Her skin had a ruddy glow, and her features were more refined than what one might imagine to be typical of the Down Syndrome stereotype. With her blonde hair and clear blue eyes, she was, in fact, a beautiful baby.

When Roberta was ten months old, at the insistence of a relative, I took her to a pediatrician who had served my husband's side of the family for many years. I was expecting to hear some words of encouragement, considering the significant gains Roberta had made during the past few months. I was completely unprepared for the doctor's prognosis: Due to Roberta's lack of muscle tone, it would be many years before she would be able to walk, if at all. It wasn't so much what he said as the way he said it. He spoke with a coldness and finality that left little room for optimism. I left his office feeling traumatized—all my hopes and dreams for Roberta had been shattered.

When I returned home, I put Roberta on my bed. She looked so small and helpless lying there. I felt sorry for her and for myself. A strange sensation of heaviness and weariness began to overpower me. Then, suddenly, all my negative thoughts and feelings vanished. In their place was something luminous and expansive. It was as if the sun had risen, shedding its victorious light over the entire earth and dispelling every type of darkness. I heard myself saying to Roberta, "You will walk, and you will be as capable as other children!" And as I spoke, a feeling of immense peace and strength flooded my heart.

Learning to Walk

At the end of Roberta's first year, I began to take classes at a yoga school in Belo Horizonte. At home I would practice near Roberta without calling attention to myself; experience had proven this to be the best method. She would watch and sometimes join in, especially with the two breathing exercises, which were her favorites. These two pranayama practices help to clean and decongest the respiratory system. They were particularly beneficial for Roberta, who had suffered from bronchial problems since birth. Roberta's daily yoga routine now included the "Spinal Twist," as well as a number of leg-strengthening exercises that had been inspired by my recent visit to the pediatrician.

Generally speaking, Roberta did asanas only with my help. She was often unwilling to initiate anything on her own and preferred having things done for her by others. This is, in fact, quite common with children who have Down Syndrome. I understood this tendency and countered it with patience and forbearance. I knew that Roberta had her own rhythm, and sooner or later she would come around.

I paid attention to every detail with Roberta and in a short time noticed that she was more observant than I had originally thought. Once, while I was doing a headstand, she took her favorite doll and placed it upside-down, leaning it against the wall. I marveled at this and imagined that one day she would be performing this posture with her own body, and not just with a toy doll.

Roberta always liked to sit cross-legged on the floor. Her favorite postures were the "Lotus Pose" and the "Easy Pose." The "Lotus Pose" locks the legs together by placing the right foot on the left thigh and the left foot on the right thigh. In the "Easy Pose," the bent legs are placed on the floor with the calf of one leg in front of the calf of the other. She would often sit in one of these two postures, lean her trunk forward, and then sleep in that position for hours. I would stretch her legs out, hoping to relieve any possible cramping, but some time later would find her cross-legged again. Finally, I decided not to interfere. It was evident that she felt comfortable sleeping this way. Moreover, these postures aid in stretching and strengthening the nerves and joints of the legs, so it was possible that Roberta was gaining some unforeseen benefit from her unusual practice.

In her sixteenth month Roberta began to walk on her own. By this time she was already able to perform many of the asanas without my help.

Preschool Years

By the time she was three, Roberta was quite mobile, though still rather lethargic. I enrolled her in a school for children with mild to severe mental retardation. Of the several special education institutions that I had investigated in Belo Horizonte, IDEC (Instituto para Desenvolvimento da Criança)[1] seemed to have the best program and atmosphere.

I remember well Roberta's first day at preschool. She cried as I started to leave her, and did not want to let go of my hand. Perhaps it was the number of students, many of them bigger than she, that frightened her. Also, at a school of this type, one may come across cases of mental and physical impairment shocking even to an adult, not to mention a child of three. For the first month she cried and whined every morning on our way to school. After that, she got used to the routine and stopped complaining.

Within a year after entering IDEC, Roberta could form sentences and hold conversations. I was working most days as a yoga teacher at the same yoga school where I had started my training. After work I would return home and help my daughters with their homework. Then the three of us would play and do yoga together.

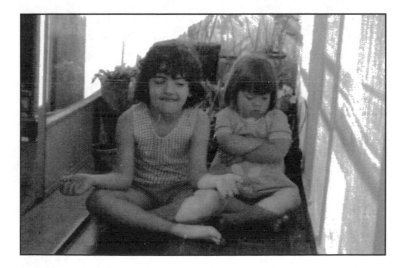

Roberta (on right) at age two and Renata (age four)

---

[1] Institute for Children's Development

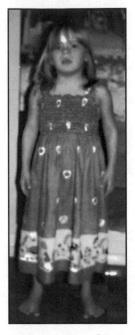

Roberta (age five)

Roberta had made great strides in her yoga practice. It was no longer necessary to lead her through any of the asana body movements. She was now working on perfecting the "Shoulder Stand," one of the inverted postures. Also, two new areas of practice had been added to her daily yoga routine: standing postures and eye exercises. The standing postures help to improve balance and leg strength, while the eye exercises develop eye movement coordination and tone the eye muscles and optic nerves. Roberta had suffered from occasional strabismus (crossed eyes) since infancy, and it was my hope that the eye exercises would help her with this problem.

After the principal at IDEC became acquainted with Roberta and learned about my therapeutic work using yoga, she invited me to teach yoga at her school. I accepted for two reasons: It would give me the opportunity to share my experience of yoga with other children at IDEC and their parents; also, it would reduce Roberta's tuition. I had recently separated from my husband and was struggling to make ends meet. Special education schools are very expensive, and by exchanging services with IDEC, I could save money.

For the next three years while Roberta attended IDEC, I continued to give yoga classes there, working primarily with children who had Down Syndrome, but also with children who had other types of disabilities. It was a "hands-on" teaching experience that helped me to validate the results of my work with Roberta. I gained many valuable insights and saw how helpful yoga was in almost every case.

During this time remarkable development in Roberta's communication and comprehension skills took place. She and Renata had become the best of friends and played together every day. Both of them enjoyed playing cards and many other educational games available in our home. Dancing was another favorite pastime. Sometimes I would put a record of popular Brazilian music on the phonograph, and hours would fly by as the three of us sang and danced together. Several times a week, I accompanied the girls to the local swim club, where we spent the early hours of the morning together. Both took swimming lessons, but while Renata was soon able to swim, it took Roberta several years longer to learn.

On weekends we often went on outings to see films and plays or to visit parks. I never tortured myself by comparing Roberta with her older sister or with other children playing in the park. From my point of view, Roberta was no different than any other child. She had certain limitations, but these limitations did not even begin to define who she was as a human being. Roberta also had many strengths, and in her own simple and unpretentious way, I think she was happier than many other children her age.

I knew there were some parents who did not agree with my way of thinking. I believe that everyone is entitled to his or her own opinion. Sometimes, however, a parent said or did something that negatively influenced their children against Roberta. The unfortunate result was that Roberta was excluded from the children's games and activities or suffered some other form of ostracism. Once, at the swim club, I saw a mother pointing at Roberta and overheard her telling her children to "be careful with your toys" and not to play with my daughter because she was a "mongoloid." Thankfully, such incidents were rare. In fact, most parents and playmates enjoyed Roberta's company because she was such an easy-going and gregarious child.

One day Renata came home feeling upset because her neighborhood friends had been laughing at her little sister. They had told her that Roberta had a silly face, with her mouth always hanging open. We had a long talk, and I tried to explain to Renata how people sometimes say hurtful things without realizing how much pain they are causing. Roberta would surely improve if we gave her our full support and loved her just the way she was. Renata was very understanding, and from then on she became my faithful assistant. Never again was she disturbed by what other people said about her sister.

In her fifth year, Roberta decided to become a vegetarian. I had stopped eating meat shortly after her birth, but continued to prepare it for my daughters, convinced that it would not be right to force my views on them. I did, however, have one rule of the house: no white sugar. This is not to say that my daughters were not allowed to eat sweets; only that I never used white sugar in my own cooking or baking.

I loved to cook and always enjoyed preparing new recipes for my family. Roberta's favorites were mashed potatoes, any dish that contained squash or cauliflower, and a special roll, very popular in our region of Brazil, called cheesebread. She used to say that I made the best cheesebread in the whole world and sometimes jokingly told me, "Oh Mom, I just ate twenty-five of your cheesebreads. They were so good!"

Roberta liked most fruits, but her favorites were bananas and tangerines, because it was easy to peel them. Homemade yogurt, eggs, and whole-wheat bread were also a regular part of her diet, as well as the high-protein combination of brown rice and beans, a staple at our house. As a matter of fact, Roberta liked almost everything I served her, with the exception of raw salads and sweets.

When we ate out, Roberta ordered french fries, or a baked potato when possible, and fresh fruit juice instead of a soft drink. Sometimes we stopped at the local ice cream parlor across the street from our swim club. Roberta always refused to order since nothing sweet really appealed to her. I could rarely resist the natural flavors of this ice cream parlor's delicious homemade ice cream and often ordered a cone. I can still recall the quizzical looks from passers-by as I walked down the street licking my double-dip cone, with Roberta empty-handed at my side.

Roberta's eating habits must have paid off, because she never had a single cavity or any other problem with her teeth or gums, something quite rare for a child with Down Syndrome. Her eyesight was also excellent. Even her strabismus eventually cleared up, according to the ophthalmologist who examined her at the age of ten. I credit this gain to the combination of eye exercises and good diet, including a daily intake of fresh fruit and vegetable juices that I substituted for the salads she never ate.

Left: Roberta with strabismus (age six). Right: Roberta doing eye exercises

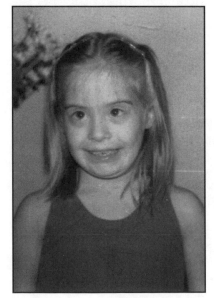
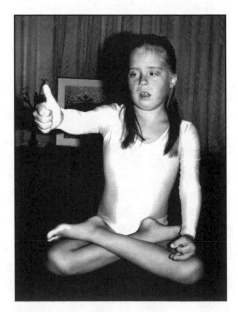

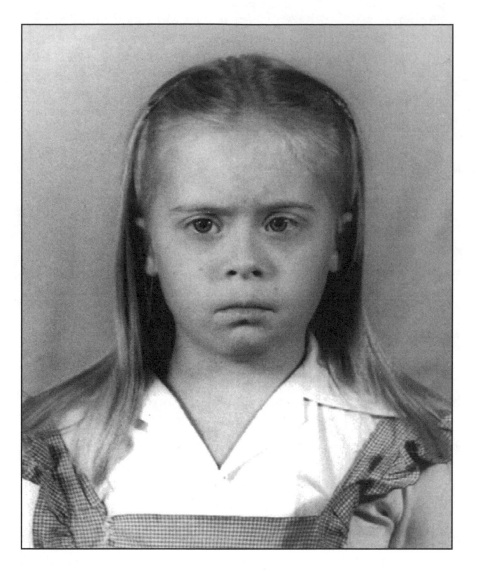

Roberta's school photo (age seven)

Getting Accepted

When Roberta was seven years old, we were able to fulfill a long-standing dream of mine. She was accepted into the local public school where her older sister Renata was studying. Her teacher at IDEC had encouraged us to apply, since Roberta was so far ahead of the rest of her class at this time. At the public school, we were fortunate to encounter an open-minded principal willing to help us with Roberta's admission.

Roberta took all the entrance tests and earned good marks, making us very excited and happy. As a result of her test scores, Roberta was assigned to a regular class. At first she found it easy to keep up with her class, but in the second semester she began to fall behind. Her areas of greatest difficulty were the basic three "R's" (reading, writing, and arithmetic). Roberta could read and write on a very rudimentary level, but her inability to master these skills affected her performance in other subjects, such as geography and history. She finished the school year with a low grade average and was assigned to a class of slower students for the following year.

In January of 1980, during Roberta's summer vacation and shortly before her eighth birthday, I opened my own yoga school in Belo Horizonte. It was a natural step in my evolution as a yoga teacher, considering the many letters and phone calls I had received inquiring about my therapy for children with special needs. Having my own center would allow me greater freedom to develop my own methods and style of teaching, which I felt was so important for the success of yoga therapy. Very soon I had a thriving yoga school where students with special needs were practicing yoga together in the same classes with my other yoga students. I also offered individual instruction for babies and children not yet ready to join a group class.

During her second year of public school, Roberta continued to experience difficulties and, despite all our efforts, was unable to finish the year with passing grades. It was a frustrating situation, and I realized that she really did need a more specialized learning environment than our public school system could offer. Nevertheless, in public school she had made great strides at the social and communicative levels and had come to feel more confident and self-reliant among children her own age.

We began to search for another special education school. I had heard about one called IBEC (Instituto Brasileiro Eduardo Claparede),[2] which had a good reputation, offering classes for children with psychomotor and social problems. I met with the school principal, who explained that their school was not structured to accommodate children with developmental disabilities. Roberta would first have to undergo a series of independent tests to determine her eligibility for acceptance. She completed the tests, and when the school staff reviewed the results, they were

---

[2] Eduardo Claparede Institute of Brazil

incredulous. Although Roberta exhibited the physical characteristics of Down Syndrome, her tests showed no further evidence of this condition.

The school administration decided to admit Roberta on probation, but requested that she repeat all the tests at IBEC, after which the principal issued the following report:

In the beginning of 1981, a mongoloid female applied for enrollment in the first grade (second grade by U.S. standards) of our elementary school, IBEC (Instituto Brasileiro Eduardo Claparede), a special education school for children and adolescents who possess a normal I.Q., but have some form of psychomotor and/or social behavior problem. In view of the fact that the applicant was a mongoloid phenotype, we turned her down because our school does not specialize in children with Down Syndrome. However, since the results of her psychological tests were surprisingly good, we asked for a period of routine observation (sensorial, motile, intellectual, emotional, and social aspects) and a possible revision of the interpretation of the tests. On one hand, we had to evaluate the organic evidence of a neurological syndrome and a previous diagnosis of mongolism—and, on the other hand, the results of a multi-dimensional examination performed by our specialized staff over a period of ninety days.

The results were the following:

- Psychiatric, Psychological, Phonological, Social Behavior, and Learning Ability Tests: good results, nearly normal development for her age.

- IQ: 87, slight mental retardation, approximately two years behind others of her age group [Down Syndrome IQ's normally range from 20 to 55].

- Language Difficulty: transposition of the phonemes /l/ and /r/ within the word.

- Sociability: has difficulty in communicating with classmates, but has good relationship with adults.

- Family Environment: has good relationship with and receives support from her mother and sister; father absent.

- Learning Capability: Although slow in her development, Roberta is both receptive and educable. She is ready to learn to read and write. She pays attention, displays interest, and demonstrates good reasoning and comprehension. Her school behavior is good, and she is progressing in all areas. Addressing the controversy between "to be and to seem" and "to seem and to be," we will not here conclude that mongolism can be cured or overcome. We would say, however, in accordance with Helene Antipoff,[3] that hers is a case of civilized intelligence; in other words, a favorable environment has helped Roberta develop her potential. This is certainly due, among other social and cultural factors, to the teaching work performed by her mother through yoga since the child's birth and, above all, to the mother's expectations of and relationship with her daughter.

Growing Up

By her tenth birthday, Roberta had successfully completed one year at IBEC, and the future looked brighter than ever. The girls and I were now a close-knit family. Renata and I continued to offer our support to Roberta, encouraging her to meet life's challenges, yet respecting her limitations. I also acknowledged my own shortcomings and limitations to Roberta to help her understand that no one is perfect.

Math was Roberta's most difficult subject in school, and she often came to me for advice when she was frustrated with her homework. One day she came home feeling particularly discouraged, and we sat down to talk. I explained to her that everyone has difficulties with one subject or another. Math had also been my most difficult subject in school, but I was finally able to master it with a little extra patience and perseverance. I put my arm around Roberta and gave her a big hug, reassuring her that everything would turn out okay if she just continued to apply herself.

Roberta and I had many conversations like this one, and I always encouraged her to pursue her goals with confidence and enthusiasm. I firmly believed that if she could apply this principle in her daily life, then sooner or later she would certainly succeed.

At this time I worked weekdays at my yoga school and traveled to other states in Brazil on weekends to conduct seminars and training courses. Returning home from work in the late

---

[3] Helene Antipoff was a famous Brazilian educator and psychologist known for her pioneering work with learning and developmental disabilities. She founded a special education school in Belo Horizonte in 1934.

afternoon, I would often be welcomed by my daughters with a short drama, which, over the years, has become etched in my memory. Entering my house, I would be greeted by Renata at the door, with Roberta conspicuously absent. "Where's Roberta?" I would ask. Renata would respond with a cryptic, "I don't know." I would begin to search the house, all the while lamenting, "Oh, where is my dear daughter? Who has taken my daughter? Where has she gone?" Suddenly, Roberta would jump out from her hiding place with an exalted, "I'm here, Mom!" and run into my arms, where we would celebrate our reunion with many hugs and kisses.

Roberta's second year at IBEC turned out to be more difficult than her first, and her third year she failed. The vice-principal called me in for a meeting and suggested that I look for another school, since it was her opinion that Roberta had already attained her optimum level of performance there. As she spoke, I began to feel a lump in my throat and was unable to respond. Somehow it just didn't seem fair that they wouldn't give my daughter a second chance.

I walked out of the vice-principal's office dreading the task that lay ahead of me. How could I tell Roberta that she had just been dismissed from IBEC without destroying her motivation and self-confidence? How could I prevent the anguish and suffering that would certainly follow? I understood that there are times when truth must be sacrificed for the sake of mercy. On my way home, I kept thinking about what I would say.

That evening I spoke with my daughters, first with Renata because she had become my confidante, and then with both together. I told Renata all that had transpired in the vice-principal's office and shed many tears. Later that evening, after regaining my composure, the three of us talked. First I told them that Roberta's final marks for the year had not been sufficient for her to advance to the next grade level at IBEC. Then I explained to Roberta that, due to the difficulty and expense involved in taking her to school every day, I thought it would be better for her to transfer to a school nearer our home.

Roberta and I began to search for another school. We applied to various educational institutions, and Roberta took their required entrance exams. It always turned out that she was either over-qualified at special education schools or under-qualified at regular education schools. Some of the principals were quite candid with me. Due to widespread prejudice and misunderstanding about Down Syndrome, they were afraid that Roberta's presence would cause their schools to lose students.

Both Renata and Roberta always liked studying, and they did their homework on their own. Roberta was not pleased with the idea of giving up her studies and just doing arts and crafts or painting. She said she was willing to participate in extracurricular activities, but she refused to stop studying.

Tired and frustrated by so many repeated rejections, I finally decided to give Roberta classes at home. I set up a classroom with a blackboard in my house, and Renata and I began to teach Roberta. We worked enthusiastically for a whole year, and the results were encouraging. Roberta's handwriting and reading comprehension improved steadily, as did her level of general knowledge.

Both my daughters helped at my yoga school in the afternoons and evenings. Roberta enjoyed being the receptionist. She would sit at my desk in the reception room studying, and when someone came to her with a question, she would provide all the necessary information in a polite and friendly manner. Roberta was able to take the bus on her own by this time, so I would often send her on simple errands, such as paying bills, cashing checks, or making small purchases.

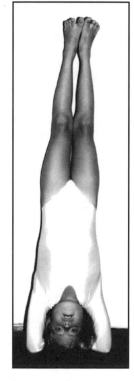

Doing the
"Headstand"

Little by little, Roberta was becoming more capable and independent. Almost every day, she and Renata practiced yoga in my adult classes, as well as in my children's classes. Roberta was now able to perform all the basic asanas and pranayama, including the "Headstand" (against a wall), not to mention some of the more difficult standing and balancing poses. She and Renata frequently accompanied me when I traveled to lecture at yoga conferences and workshops. As part of my presentation, each of my daughters would perform a choreography of yoga asanas which she had created by herself and rehearsed beforehand. I was so proud of both my daughters and amazed by the grace and precision with which Roberta flowed from one posture to another in her "dance" of yoga.

During the publication party for the first edition of *Yoga for the Special Child* in November of 1983, Roberta was there with me, both of us giving autographs side by side. She was so exuberant and self-confident that she even congratulated me on having written "her book."

I had known for some time that it was my daughter's dream to be a yoga teacher when she grew up. In a recent conversation with another yoga student, Roberta had stated that she wanted to teach other children everything she had learned from her mother when she "had been Down," as she used to refer to her condition. In her own mind, Roberta was no longer disabled.

Despite Roberta's significant accomplishments and the remarkable change in her physical features, she still felt sad and out of place when she heard other people talking about school. On these occasions I tried to console her, explaining that though we hadn't found a school this year, we would surely find one next year.

And that's what actually happened. In January of 1985 we found the ideal school, a special education institute called INAPLIC (Instituto de Aplicação Biopsicologica).[4] The principal and all the staff were sensitive and competent. Roberta felt at ease there and liked her teachers and classmates. She worked hard and continued to progress, expanding her potential and moving ever closer toward achieving the success and happiness I had promised her in the hospital, shortly after her birth.

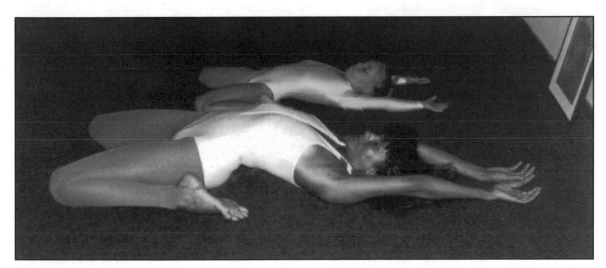

Mother and daughter practicing yoga together

---

[4] Institute for the Application of Biopsychology

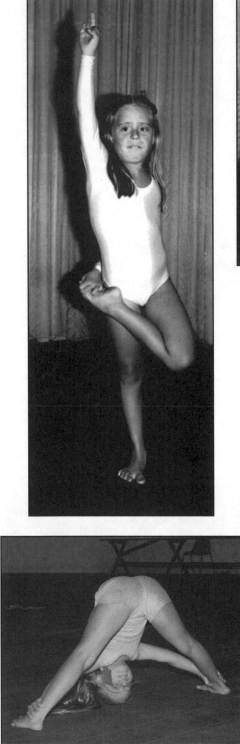

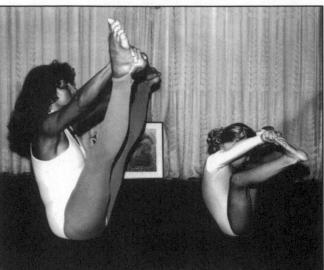

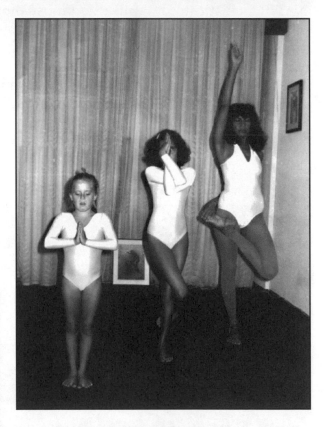

Clockwise from upper left: Roberta performing a standing pose (age nine); practicing yoga with her mother; practicing together with her sister and mother; performing a standing forward-bending pose at an international yoga conference.

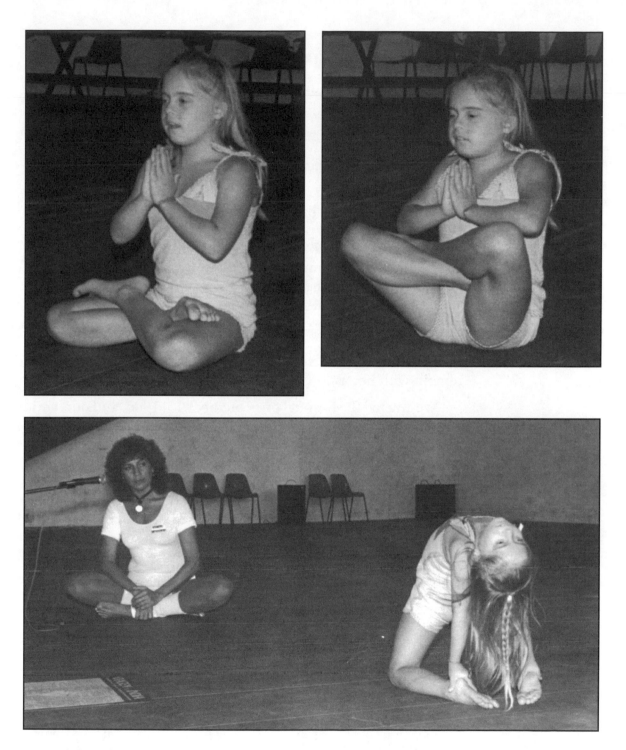

Upper left and right: Roberta performing at an international yoga conference. Below: Roberta and her mother at the same conference. Her mother is seated at the microphone explaining the therapeutic effects of the asanas that Roberta is performing.

Mission Accomplished

In December of 1985, when Roberta was thirteen years old, she began to experience various health problems. At first she appeared tired, listless, and slower in her movements and reflexes; then she began to gain weight. I took her to several doctors, but the cause of her problems remained a mystery.

Nine months later, she contracted a non-specific viral infection, accompanied by high fever and swelling of the lymph nodes, and needed to be hospitalized. She was frightened by the prospect of staying alone in the hospital, so I made arrangements with the hospital staff to rent a private room which Renata and I could share with her. Because children with Down Syndrome are generally more susceptible to infectious disease and do not respond well to medication, no one could project the length of Roberta's hospital stay. Thanks to the compassionate financial assistance of my concerned yoga students and their families, I was able to remain with her as long as necessary.

We entered the hospital on September 15, 1986, and our world was suddenly reduced to a single small room. Day and night I cared for Roberta with my total love and attention, attending to her physical needs and comforting her with my words and lullabies. The strangeness of the hospital environment, exaggerated by the intensity of her illness, caused Roberta so much anxiety that she was unable to relax without my physical touch. For hours on end I massaged and stroked her fevered body to help relieve her nervousness and tension. When darkness came, I sat on the end of her bed and held her feet in my lap. Only then was she able to sleep.

During our second week together, Roberta's illness became further complicated by an infection that she contracted in the hospital. Her condition took a marked turn for the worse, and she was transferred to the intensive care unit. I continued to spend my days with Roberta in intensive care and returned late each night to our rented hospital room, where I slept with Renata, who was attending school at the time. Hoping and praying for my daughter's recovery, I remained with Roberta until our eighteenth day in the hospital, when I needed to go home to pick up some fresh clothes.

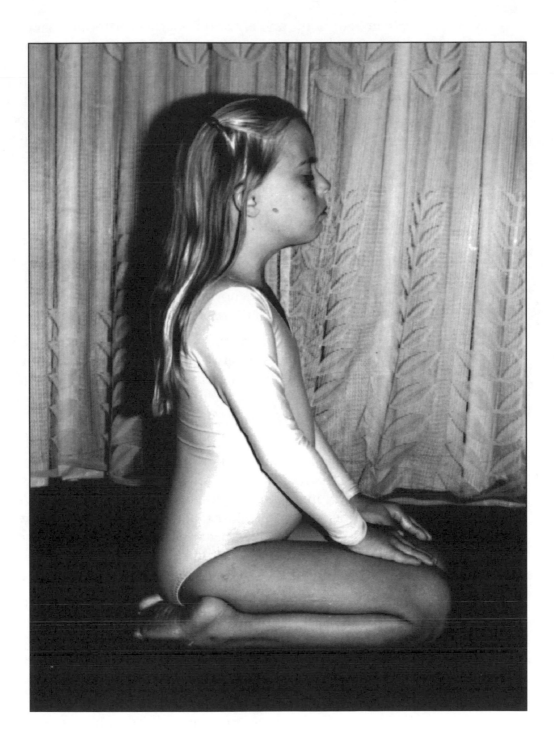

When I got home and entered Roberta's bedroom, I sat down on her bed and began to look around the room, thinking about the nightmare we were going through at the hospital. My eyes came to rest upon the step stool by her bed. All her school material was stacked neatly upon it, as she was in the habit of doing after finishing her homework. I picked up one of her notebooks and opened it. Her handwriting was so beautiful! She was so dedicated to her homework. Even her last assignment was finished and ready for school.

Suddenly I understood — Roberta's mission was already accomplished; not even her homework was left undone. She had had enough time to carry out everything she came here for, from the easiest things to the most difficult. She had overcome her physical and mental limitations. Everything was completed and finished here. What she was now undergoing in the hospital was necessary to dissolve her last ties to this earthly plane.

I returned to the hospital with our clothes and continued to care for Roberta as her strength ebbed away. Shortly after midnight on October 9, her twenty-fourth day in the hospital, Roberta passed away. Following the funeral, I took her ashes to Rio de Janeiro and offered them to the ocean.

After Roberta's death, I thought of closing my yoga school, since she had been the inspiration and focal point for my work. I recalled how Roberta had come into my life and, step by step, led the way in developing a successful therapy for children with special needs. Then it became clear that I could not allow her wonderful contribution to disappear just because she was gone. Although Roberta's mission was finished, mine was not.

Despite my grief, I knew I had to go on. I wanted to hold Roberta so badly, to feel her touch, and to receive her love again; yet Renata and many others still needed me. Somehow, I would have to alter my perspective and learn to love Roberta on a different, more subtle level in order to alleviate the almost visceral pain that I was experiencing over her physical loss.

Nowadays I see that Roberta is still with me in every child I work with. Whenever I give or receive affection from these children, I feel the same love, the same light. I no longer suffer from the emptiness of her loss because I have found in each child the reason for my life.

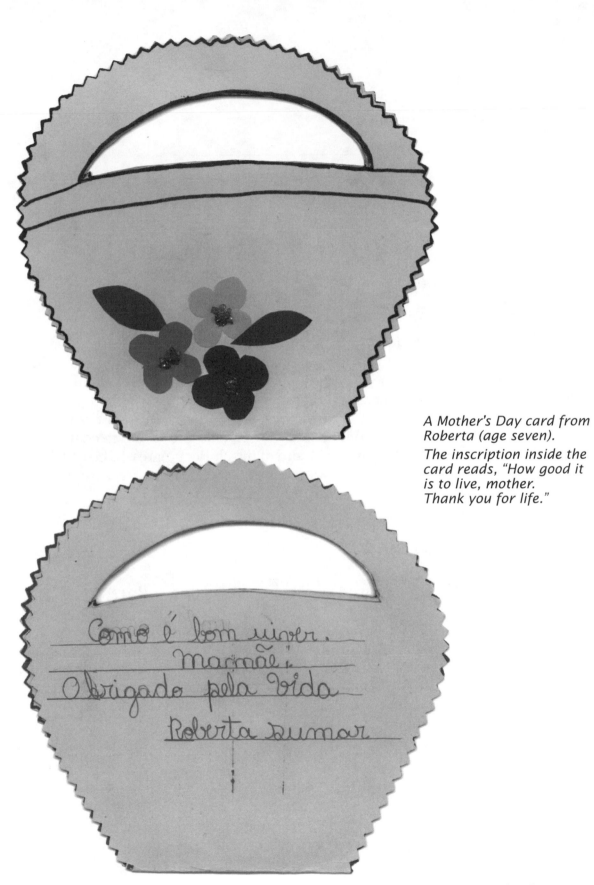

A Mother's Day card from Roberta (age seven).

The inscription inside the card reads, "How good it is to live, mother. Thank you for life."

2

Case Histories and Testimonials

The following case histories chronicle the progress of two children: one with Down Syndrome, the other with microcephaly. Each history includes a description of the child's condition according to medical examination (when this information is available), parents' observations and testimonials, and my personal evaluation. Conferences with parents and recommendations are noted, along with a record of the child's progress. The case histories are followed by a series of personal accounts, written by the parents of my students.

Mariana

Comments by Mariana's Parents

My husband and I married two years ago, and the birth of Mariana introduced us to an entirely new world. The delivery was easy, but a long time seemed to pass before Mariana was returned to our room in the hospital. We experienced many positive feelings during those first hours of her existence; she was our first daughter.

The next day we were informed by a group of doctors that Mariana showed many of the characteristics of Down Syndrome, and they had also detected a murmur in her heart. Our first reaction was feelings of doubt, uncertainty, and sadness. Then we resigned ourselves to the situation and decided to search for appropriate information and treatment.

Soon after, we heard through friends about the work of Sonia Sumar in Belo Horizonte. We found it interesting that yoga was being taught to children with special needs, and when Mariana was a month old, we enrolled her in a program of yoga therapy at Sonia's center. We also started taking lessons there, which piqued Mariana's interest in yoga and helped her become more receptive to her own practice. The asanas, relaxation techniques, breathing exercises, and chants that Sonia taught us changed our family environment, which is now more harmonious and calm.

The physical characteristics of Down Syndrome present at birth diminished as time went by. Now Mariana has an expressive face, a bright look, and an ever-present smile. She eats well and sleeps soundly. At no time has she had a serious problem with her health.

She is now thirteen months old and is crawling all over the house. She walks with assistance and likes to ride in the car and visit shopping centers. For her age, she is affectionate and clever, learns quickly, and has a fundamental grasp of how and why things work. Most important, the heart murmur has disappeared.

According to her pediatrician, Mariana's development is nearly normal. We believe that her remarkable progress is the result of Sonia's program of yoga therapy. Sonia's work is done with love— a love that embraces her fellow human beings just as they are, with all their limitations. She receives everybody with open arms and an open heart. Her work is serious, beautiful, and filled with sincere emotion. Knowing her has been a great help to us in our daily lives.

Finally, we can say that Mariana has taught us many things, made us meet very special people, and put us in touch with a whole new world. That is why we are so proud of her and satisfied with her accomplishments.

Juarez Andrade Tolentino and Eliana Tolentino
Belo Horizonte, November 17, 1991

My Comments

Born by Caesarean section on September 29, 1990, in Belo Horizonte, Mariana is the elder of two sisters in the Tolentino family. I met Mariana and her parents, Juarez and Eliana, in November, when she was one month old. After an evaluation of Mariana and a consultation with her parents, she and both parents enrolled in my yoga school and began taking classes there. Each of the parents participated in two adult classes per week, and Mariana attended two 30-minute yoga therapy sessions per week.

My work with Mariana started out rather slowly due to her congenital heart problem. According to her pediatrician, the murmur required corrective surgery, so I had to be especially careful not to stress Mariana's heart in any of the postures or exercises. One basic precautionary measure was to provide her with rest periods whenever she appeared to be tiring. Another measure, even more important, was not to place her in any of the inverted postures. Any movement that raised both her lower trunk and legs above the chest, thereby increasing the pressure within the heart, might aggravate her problem.

My approach was to strengthen Mariana's heart and circulatory system through a series of preparatory exercises and postures that were totally safe for her to practice. As she gradually improved, I could increase the duration of these exercises and add more difficult ones. The objective was to stimulate her development by helping her expand her limits, yet never going beyond these limits at any one time. This type of therapeutic work is painstaking and delicate, requiring sensitivity on the part of the yoga therapist and a thorough attunement with the child.

In addition to a heart problem (which occurs in approximately forty percent of all children with Down Syndrome), Mariana presented many of the characteristic Down Syndrome features. These included hypotonia (low muscle tone), a flattened nose and midface, low placement of the ears, and slightly slanted eyes with epicanthal folds of skin at the inner corners. In order to help her overcome the hypotonia and prepare her body for the practice of asanas, I incorporated many muscle strengthening exercises in her yoga routine. Key areas to strengthen were the muscles of her neck, arms, feet, legs, and abdomen, as well as the joints in her shoulders and hips. These exercises included leg and arm lifts, and movements that flexed the shoulders, hips, knees, ankles, and

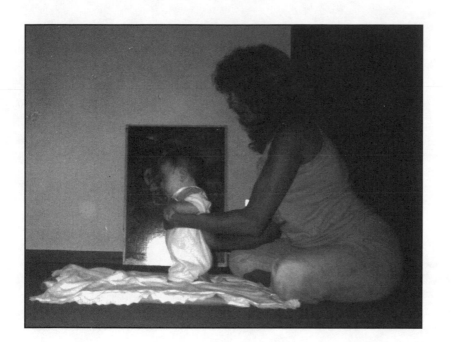

Teaching Mariana
to sit

joints of the feet. Each session ended with a ten-minute period of deep relaxation, giving Mariana's body an opportunity to absorb the benefits of all the previous exercises.

As expected, Mariana was totally passive during our initial yoga sessions. I had to perform all the movements with her body, like a puppeteer who pulls the strings attached to the different parts of a marionette in order to make it move. However, she improved noticeably with each session and was soon participating in all the exercises.

Right from the very start, Mariana's development took an even, uphill course. She was always calm, understanding, and receptive. I believe her steady progress was due to her parents' active participation in yoga, our consultations together, and their belief that Mariana would improve.

During the consultations I explained the various stages of development that Mariana would have to pass through, and how to set up and conduct their daughter's yoga classes at home. I always set aside time for Juarez and Eliana to ask questions, and sometimes I questioned them, especially if I had noticed a recent change in Mariana's behavior. The end result of this open communication between Mariana's parents and myself was that they were able to create a more supportive home environment, which included weekly yoga classes taught by one of the parents.

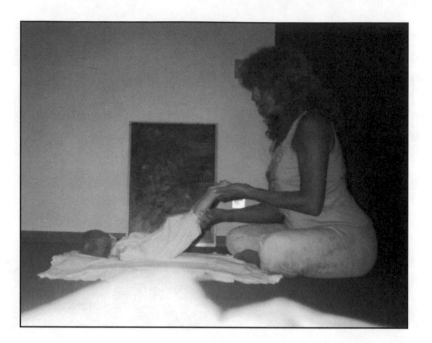

Performing the "Locust Pose"

At Mariana's monthly medical examination, her pediatrician was always surprised by the vast improvement in her since the previous checkup. This encouraged me to experiment with more advanced exercises and postures, which I always monitored closely to make sure that her response was positive. However, I never included these advanced exercises in the routines which I designed for Mariana at home.

At eight months, Mariana was able to sit on her own; at nine months, to crawl; and at ten months, to stand alone. With the achievement of each new milestone, I was able to add new poses to her yoga routine. These included the "Spinal Twist" and variations of the "Forward-Bending Pose" (all of which begin from a sitting position), and several standing poses (which begin with the child on her feet). The standing poses develop equilibrium and strengthen the muscles of the legs and lower back. They are an important aid in preparing a young child to walk. During this same period, I also introduced one of the yogic breathing exercises, the "Cleansing Breath." However, as is the case with many children her age, Mariana just watched me and smiled each time I demonstrated this exercise to her.

In Mariana's eleventh month, her pediatrician examined her and was unable to detect any sign of a heart murmur. This was a great triumph for all of us, and a great relief to know that Mariana no longer needed surgery. Now I could finally begin to work with the inverted postures. These poses are especially beneficial for any child with a nervous system dysfunction because of their powerful effect on the sense organs, brain, and upper endocrine glands.[1]

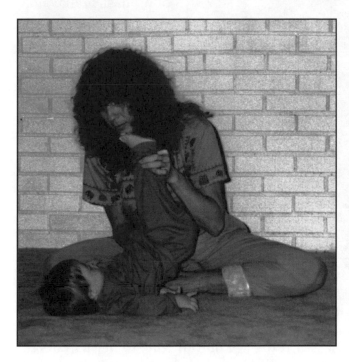 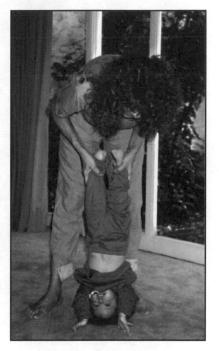

Left: Performing the "Shoulder Stand"
Right: Performing the "Headstand"

As she continued to progress in her development, I often tested Mariana by placing her in a standing position, back against the wall, and coaxing her to come to me. I knew that she possessed the necessary strength and balance to walk because she was now performing several of the standing poses without any assistance on my part. Then one day, during a yoga session, I placed her against the wall and she took three wobbly steps. This was in her sixteenth month. After the session, when I saw Eliana, I told her that she was in store for a pleasant surprise. That same evening she called me back with the good news that Mariana had taken her first steps at home.

In Mariana's eighteenth month, I decided to place her in a group yoga class with other children. She had already mastered all the basic poses, performing most of them without any assistance on my part. Now it was time for her to move on to a more independent type of practice, which would help her to develop greater com-

---

[1] The thyroid, parathyroid, pituitary, and pineal glands.

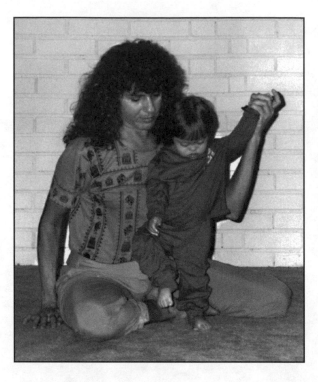

Attempting the "Tree Pose"

munication and socialization skills, in addition to refining and expanding her practice of asanas, pranayama, and deep relaxation.

Today, Mariana is a healthy, happy, well-adjusted child of six. She attends regular classes at a public school and is doing well in all her subjects. Her diction is excellent, and she socializes well with her schoolmates and friends. She rides a bicycle, dresses and cares for herself, and loves to dance. She has a good relationship with her younger sister, and participates in all the activities and social events that her school friends do. Despite the fact that Mariana discontinued formal yoga classes at the age of four (due to her parents relocating to another neighborhood), it is clear that her three years of practice have held her in good stead.

Her Pediatrician's Testimonial

I declare that little Mariana Tolentino has been my patient since the gestation period. Down Syndrome was verified at delivery by her hypotonia and other characteristic features. In her second month, she began a program of yoga therapy, with accompanying stimulatory exercises provided by her parents at home.

During her first year of life, Mariana showed no sign of a delay in her development. However, what surprised us most, along with the strengthening of her muscles, were some physical alterations, such as the shifting of her ears from a low to normal position in her head. Another physical alteration, even more noteworthy, was the complete disappearance of her heart murmur, which we had believed could only be corrected through surgery.

Gláucia Maria Moreira Galvão, M.D.
(Mariana's pediatrician)
Belo Horizonte, October 21, 1991

Photos of Mariana at Various Ages

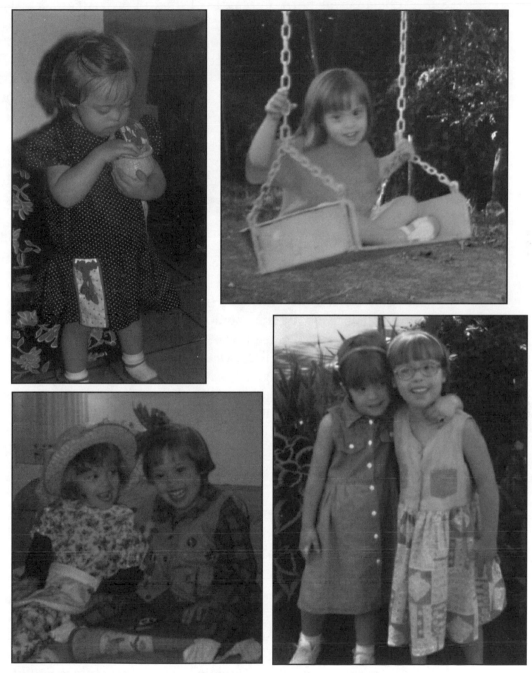

Top left: Mariana at her second birthday Top right: At three years
Bottom left: Party time! Mariana (on right) at age four with her sister
Isabela (age two) Bottom right: At age five with Isabela

Luciana

Luciana was born on May 14, 1980 in Porto Alegre, a coastal city in the southernmost region of Brazil. Delivered prematurely by emergency Caesarean section, Luciana weighed 6½ pounds and measured 19½ inches. Her mother, Valderez, soon noticed abnormalities, such as restricted movements, weak suckling, and complete lack of crying. When she asked the pediatrician's opinion, however, she was told these behavioral deficits were all in her imagination.

Several days after returning home, Luciana stopped breathing. Valderez gave her mouth-to-mouth resuscitation until they were able to reach the nearest hospital. After three months of medical evaluation, the doctors finally gave Valderez a diagnosis of her daughter's condition: vegetative microcephaly, probably caused by fetal distress due to lack of oxygen at the time of birth.

I first met Luciana and Valderez in September of 1982 at a yoga school in Porto Alegre, where I had been invited to attend a seminar and speak about the therapeutic methods described in my book. At this time Luciana was two years old and weighed 26½ pounds. She was hemiplegic (paralyzed on one side of the body), hypotonic (lacking muscle tone), hyposensitive (partially insensitive to pain), semi-strabismic (cross-eyed), and exhibited stereotyped head movements (hitting her head against walls or floors). She had already had six respiratory arrests, two cardiac arrests, twelve hospitalizations, and countless convulsions. In addition, she was unable to ingest solids and received anti-convulsive medication daily.

Discouraged by the poor results of medical treatment to date, Valderez asked me if yoga could help her child. I told her I had never worked with this condition, but added that my confidence in yoga led me to believe it might indeed help.

Feedback from this seminar was so positive that a month later I returned to Porto Alegre to start a course for children with disabilities. Over the next year, I conducted workshops one weekend each month, consisting of two full days of instruction and practice. The time was divided equally between the children and their parents. Although Valderez lived outside Porto Alegre proper and suffered severe financial hardships, she decided to enroll Luciana, for which she received a substantial reduction in class fees.

The course began in November of 1981, with a focus on respiration. I explained how proper diaphragmatic breathing helped to oxygenate the blood and strengthen the nervous system. Later, I demonstrated to Valderez and the other participants the method for teaching diaphragmatic breathing to infants, and then assisted as they repeated my movements with their children. We included one pranayama practice, the "Cleansing Breath," to clear the upper and lower respiratory tracts.

To prepare Luciana for the practice of asanas, I guided her body through a number of muscle-strengthening and body-awareness exercises, including movements of the arms, legs, feet, and head. The entire class consisted of three segments: five minutes for breathing practices, fifteen minutes for body movements and asanas, and ten minutes for relaxation practices.

In addition to the above exercises and practices, I covered a number of other topics, including diet and nutrition, chromotherapy (exposure to different colored lights), and the use of affirmations. I also talked about the importance of the parents' attitude toward their child, and explained how to create a positive learning environment at home.

Valderez's receptivity was a great aid in my work with Luciana. Sometimes she would spend a whole month teaching Luciana a single breathing practice and posture. I had explained to her that each exercise, no matter how simple it seemed, would bring about powerful changes in her daughter's physical and mental makeup. Luciana's two older sisters also offered cooperation and support. As a result, each time I arrived in Porto Alegre on my monthly visit, I found Luciana greatly improved.

Within three months of beginning yoga therapy, Luciana had made remarkable progress in her ability to communicate with others. She was nursing well and even eating with a spoon, though still unable to chew solid foods.

I felt myself being drawn closer and closer to Luciana and her family. During my absence they wrote often, keeping me informed throughout the month. Valderez filled out and returned the questionnaire that I had provided to each of the participants in the course. This helped me to plan my upcoming program for Luciana. She also sent photographs demonstrating Luciana's progress and development. Gains could be seen in Luciana's facial expression; her formerly vague and lusterless look had changed to a bright and attentive one.

After four months, I began teaching her sitting exercises with forward-bending and twisting movements. Later, I added inverted postures, to help bring fresh blood to the brain and to tone the nervous system. Little by little, Luciana began to acquire a better command and knowledge of her body, obviously delighted with her new-found abilities.

By her sixth month of treatment, Luciana no longer needed diapers. Her ability to communicate through body language and verbalization had taken a quantum leap. In response to her development, I continued to apply increasingly complex exercises, many of which she learned to perform on her own. In her seventh month, she was able to stand without support.

By October of 1983, one year after the course had begun, all convulsions had ceased. Luciana could walk by herself, travel up and down stairs, and open and close doors. She laughed, danced, and played with the family dog. All these wonderful developments had taken place because Valderez had chosen to work for her daughter's rehabilitation, rather than to believe the doctors who had told her that Luciana was a "hopeless" case.

The human mind is indeed difficult to fathom. A physician can diagnose a child as brain-damaged, but the extent of this damage and the chances of achieving some degree of functional development and socialization, time and effort can alone decide. Besides, much of a child's progress in rehabilitation therapy depends on the parents' attitude toward their child and their willingness to trust in the efficacy of the program.

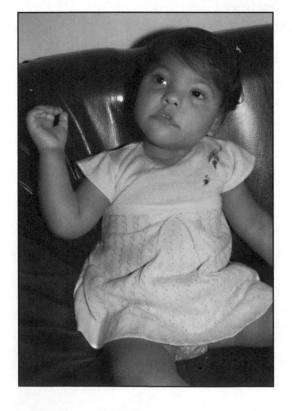

Luciana after four months of yoga therapy. She still could not sit on her own.

When the course ended in Porto Alegre, I was grateful to have had the opportunity to work with Luciana and her mother. The family continued to write me for some time. Later, they moved away, and I no longer had the opportunity to visit them regularly. Then we lost touch.

In February of 1994, anxious to see how Luciana had fared over a decade, I determined to search them out. I went back to Porto Alegre and finally found them far from the center of the city. When I saw

Photos depicting Luciana's progress

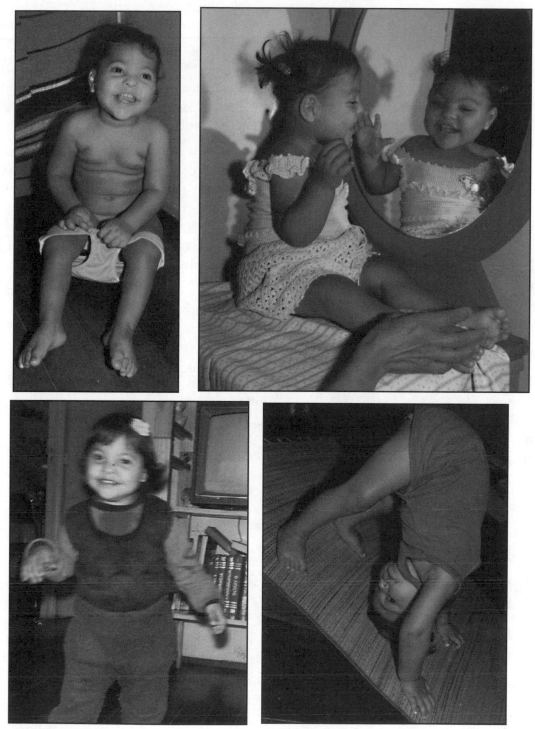

Clockwise from upper left: After five months of yoga therapy; Luciana in her sixth month of yoga therapy; practicing yoga in her ninth month of yoga therapy; Luciana after one year of yoga therapy, at the completion of the course.

Luciana, I felt a tremendous disappointment. Valderez had discontinued all treatment, including yoga exercises. Serious financial problems still beset her, and she had run out of incentive to improve her family's situation.

Luciana had regressed pitiably. Though still able to walk, her posture was no longer erect. Her cognitive, communicative, and motor skills had also deteriorated. Nonverbal and aggressive, she sought attention by biting people and pulling their hair.

Valderez recounted a tale of woe about their recent years. There was little I could do by way of financial assistance or effective emotional support. I left feeling quite discouraged. In trying to help Luciana, perhaps I had not given Valderez the support she needed to overcome the obstacles in her own life. Through correspondence, I will now do my best to revive her hope and courage, so that together we may take up this work of love again.

Luciana's case demonstrates the possibility of rehabilitating a child whose condition doctors had considered irreversible. It is also a strong argument for continuing therapy, even after important developmental milestones have been reached.

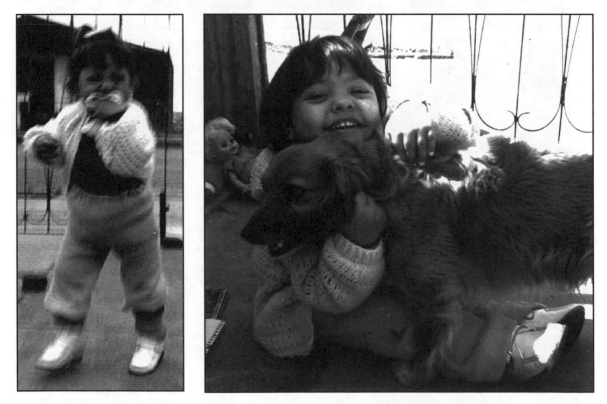

Left and Right: Luciana after one year of yoga therapy, at the completion of the course.

Letters from the Parents of My Students

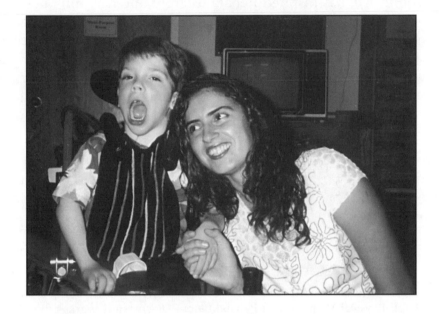

Param and Renata

I would like to share my observations about the ongoing benefits of yoga for my son, Param. He is nine years old and has severe physical limitations related to cerebral palsy. In 1995 our family was extremely fortunate to have Sonia Sumar's daughter, Renata, stay at our home in Virginia. Three days a week, for four months, Renata conducted a one-hour yoga session with Param.

The effect on his body tone was immediately noticeable. His sitting posture and sitting balance improved. His body tone relaxed, especially in the shoulders, arms, and hands, enabling him to more easily perform tasks requiring upper-extremity dexterity. His head and neck alignment improved, allowing him to hold his head erect for significantly longer periods. Cognitively, he was able to pay attention to conversations for a longer time before becoming fatigued and was more focused while listening. An integrated calmness of body and centeredness developed as the yoga therapy sessions continued. Because of the cumulative benefits of regular practice, his spinal scoliosis diminished. It also became apparent to his physician and therapists that, due to his decreased muscle tone, the surgery contemplated for Param was no longer necessary. This surgery is often performed on the muscle group that causes hip dysplasia.

I want to acknowledge and emphasize here the direct influence that Renata has had in this process. Besides being a superb yoga practitioner, she is a wonderful embodiment of the spirit of yoga. Sonia's enthusiasm for yoga, imparted to her daughter from a young age, has inspired Renata to grow into a shining person, filled with compassion, joy, and a love of service to the world. Renata is not only a gifted yoga teacher, but also a certified speech and language pathologist. As a result, she was able to give Param training in oral motor skills. His tongue-thrusting and other increased-tone symptoms were greatly reduced as a direct result of Renata's intervention.

In conclusion, I believe that Param has continued to benefit from Renata's work with him in 1995. I attribute this both to her expertise as a yoga therapist and to her integrity and dedication as a person. Thank you, Renata, for the wonderful gift you have given us.

Richard Atman Johnson, R.N., for the Johnson Family
Buckingham, Virginia, May 26, 1997

Richard Johnson has been a Registered Nurse for twelve years, specializing in Adult Physical Medicine and Rehabilitation. He currently works at the University of Virginia Medical Center.

Testimonial of Param's Physical Therapist

During a period of approximately four months, "P.J.," a nine-year-old child with severe total body dystonia and dyskinesia secondary to Cerebral Palsy, was fortunate to receive adjunctive regular yoga therapy in addition to his regular weekly combined Physical Therapy-Occupational Therapy treatment. The latter therapy consisted primarily of neuro-developmental therapy; orthopedic therapy; myofascial release techniques; and use of custom adapted positioning and mobility devices and assistive technology devices as needed.

Among the improvements noted in P.J.'s condition during this period of combined yoga and traditional PT-OT therapy were:

1. An apparent overall "quieting" of the central nervous system, with a decrease in P.J.'s tendency to thrust into total body extensor patterns; a decrease in his tendency to "generate" muscle tone through severe jaw extension; and a decrease in his tendency to "hold his breath" during strong volitional efforts.

2. A decrease in muscle tone of the upper extremities during intentional movements, allowing P.J. to more easily reach and press switches to operate a toy.

3. An increase in passive joint range of motion, particularly in the hamstrings and hip adductor-internal rotator muscles, which contributed to P.J.'s ability to sit independently on a mat cross-legged for the first time in his life.

4. An increase in P.J.'s ability to redirect attention to tasks when requested to do so; a decrease in distractibility; and an increase in eye-to-eye contact.

5. A noticeable improvement in P.J.'s breathing pattern characterized by slower, deeper breaths.

6. An improved ability for P.J. to "tune into" his own high body tone and to self-inhibit this tone.

7. An apparent improvement in self-esteem and confidence.

It certainly appeared, in P.J.'s case, that yoga therapy was a very beneficial adjunct to traditional PT and OT treatment, and that it contributed to enhancing P.J.'s physical, mental, and emotional development in a safe, gentle, and loving way.

Kathryn T. Broecker, R.T.P., M.S.
Director of Physical Therapy, Richmond Cerebral Palsy Center
Richmond, Virginia, April 21, 1997

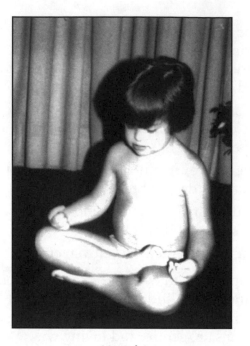

Maurício

I became involved in yoga therapy because my fourth child, Maurício, was born with Down Syndrome. Yoga practices had such a profound effect on his mental and emotional development that he was able to enter a regular preschool at the age of three. At preschool, he adjusted well to the curriculum and made friends with both the teachers and other children his age.

I see Maurício as a child with some limitations, but also with a great potential. Among other benefits, yoga has helped him develop concentration, balance, and motor coordination. In addition to yoga therapy, Maurício is involved in an early intervention program at a local clinic.

Solange Macagnnan
Cruz Alta, January 10, 1986

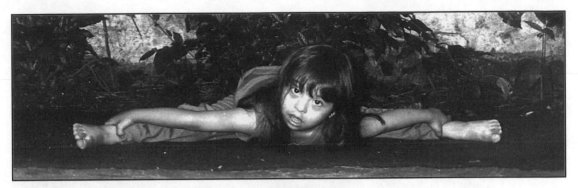

Isabela Cristina

My name is Eliane, and my five-year-old daughter, Isabela Cristina, has Down Syndrome. She began yoga therapy when she was seven months old. Since then, she has always had excellent posture and good muscle tone. Her general understanding has also improved, and her creativity and imagination have blossomed.

In order to understand the benefits of yoga, you must practice it. Yoga develops the whole person. It stimulates the cerebral areas by irrigating the brain cells with fresh blood; it balances the emotions; it fortifies the lungs and heart; and it stretches and tones the muscles. Ultimately it benefits the entire body and mind. Another thing I love about yoga is that it is not just for children with special needs. At Sonia's yoga school, students with special needs practice yoga together with her other yoga students. In this way, yoga becomes a natural setting for the process of group integration.

Isabela and I are very pleased with yoga. I hope she will never stop practicing.

Eliane da Costa
Belo Horizonte, November 15, 1991

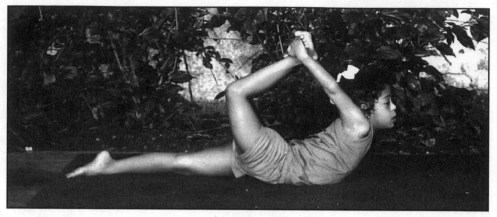
Lorena

I first learned of Sonia Sumar's yoga therapy through an article in the newspaper. I immediately felt that Sonia was the kind of person who could understand the heartache I was going through with my child. I was certain she would be able to answer all my questions, because here was a mother who had already successfully completed a journey that I was just beginning.

Now that my daughter and I have had the opportunity to experience some of the benefits of yoga practice, I thank God for that newspaper article, which led me to Sonia Sumar and her community of yoga practitioners. I say "community" in the literal sense of the word, since all of us are friends who share a common bond, and we are able to support one another through an open exchange of ideas and experiences.

Lorena began practicing yoga with Sonia in August of 1983, when she was nine months old, and now it is a part of our daily life. But yoga is not like any sport. It is much more comprehensive.

Nowadays, "Lo" is nine years old and studies at a public school near our home. It is difficult to describe the light, tranquility, strength, and optimism that yoga brings to us. My little daughter is a happy, communicative, and intelligent child. We are very proud of her.

Glória Buval Moreira
Belo Horizonte, December 1, 1991

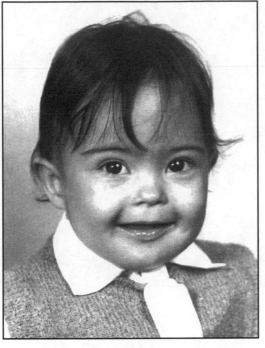

Thiago

In August of 1984 our son Thiago was born with Down Syndrome, diagnosed by the pediatrician at the hospital. My husband and I were astonished by the doctor's complete lack of understanding in explaining our son's condition to us. We were told Thiago would always be a problem, and there was nothing we could do to improve his situation.

One day, a neighbor lent me the first edition of *Yoga for the Special Child* by Sonia Sumar, which I read with great interest. Then I decided to meet with Sonia about Thiago. He was twenty days old when he began yoga therapy at her center. Sonia taught me everything I needed to know, even about natural diet and food preparation. Thiago is a year old now and does not eat meat or white sugar. He is very healthy and has never taken any medicine.

Thiago has turned out to be completely the opposite of the doctor's prognosis. He is a happy and clever child. He is alert, perceptive, and aware of his relationships with others. What I like most in him is the love he transmits to everybody—thanks to yoga and Sonia Sumar.

Maria Ferreira Ribeiro and Orlando Araújo Ribeiro
Belo Horizonte, December 4, 1985

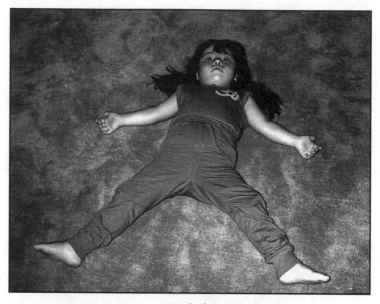

Isabela

Isabela started yoga therapy when she was five months old. Before that, we consulted with many doctors to get information on Down Syndrome. Most of them gave us a very negative prognosis. We kept on searching until we found the right person: Sonia Sumar. After evaluating Isabela, Sonia gave us a hopeful outlook for the first time, showing us light where there had only been darkness. During Isabela's first month of practice, we noticed a marked improvement in many areas of her development, proving the intrinsic value of yoga as a therapy for our daughter.

Now Isabela is almost four years old. She is a well-adjusted and happy child, and we are proud of her.

Araci Inácio Magalhães Giani
Belo Horizonte, November 18, 1991

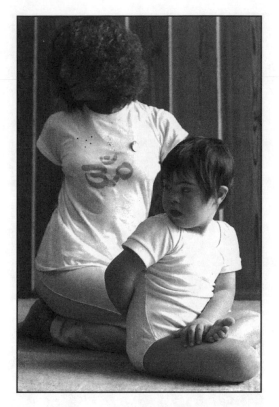

Eloísa

In a few short sentences, it would be impossible for me to re-late all that yoga has done for my daughter. Nevertheless, I would like to share my testimonial with the many mothers who are searching for a way to improve the lives of their children with Down Syndrome. Thanks to the benefits of yogic breathing exer-cises and asanas, my 3½-year-old daughter, Eloísa, is a balanced, calm, and happy child, with practically normal development for her age. She walks, talks, and knows everybody in the neighbor-hood. This year she entered a regular preschool.

We are deeply grateful to Sonia Sumar, a gifted and caring teacher.

Maria Piedade Kilson
Belo Horizonte, December 1, 1985

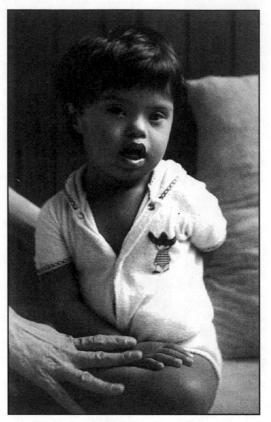

Helinho

Two years ago, my son, Helinho, began practicing yoga with Sonia Sumar. We could soon see the benefits in terms of his mental and physical development. Even the other specialists working with him were surprised by the increase in his capacity for reasoning and concentration.

Recently, Helinho underwent two surgeries and amazed us with his comprehension of the whole process, despite his three years of age. These kinds of experiences are giving mothers of children with disabilities the hope that our sons and daughters will someday be self-sufficient members of society.

Maria Luiza Resende Gomes
Belo Horizonte, November 3, 1985

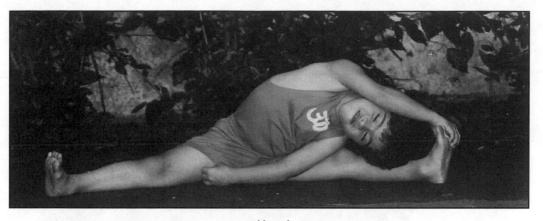

Henrique

Any parents who have the good fortune to work with Sonia Sumar are sure to see great advances in their child's development. For three years now, our son Henrique has been enjoying the benefits of yoga practice. In his daily life, he has shown noticeable improvements on both a physical and mental level.

We will always be grateful to Sonia Sumar for her dedication to helping others and for the guidance and assistance she has given us.

> *Gláucia and Aloísio Magalhães*
> Belo Horizonte, November 12, 1991

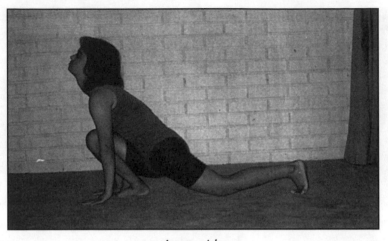

Aparecida

Aparecida has been practicing yoga at Sonia's center for seven years now, and during this time we have seen one improvement after another. Her breathing is deep and regular, and her body is balanced and beautiful. She is always calm and easygoing. Yoga has been the best thing in her life, and she is crazy about her teacher and classes. At the center, she receives only encouragement. We are very pleased with Aparecida's development and want to say "thank you" to Sonia Sumar.

Marieta Clélia Campos
Belo Horizonte, November 29, 1991

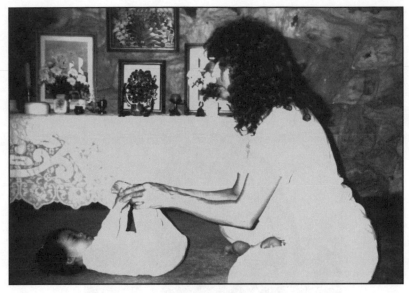

Taíza

With my daughter, Taíza, I have always tried to focus on the optimistic side of things, and to believe with all my heart in her inherent potential. In the past I investigated a number of therapies to see which one would be best suited for her. In my opinion, it is the parents' responsibility to choose the best form of therapy for their child.

Finally I found yoga, a gentle and harmonious way of exercising the body and mind. Even though my daughter and I have only been practicing yoga for a short time, we can already see excellent results. Our lives have changed on many levels, and we both feel more self-reliant and full of peace.

I am deeply grateful to Sonia Sumar, who has shared these valuable teachings with us.

Helenicé Ude Marques de Oliveira
Belo Horizonte, November 13, 1991

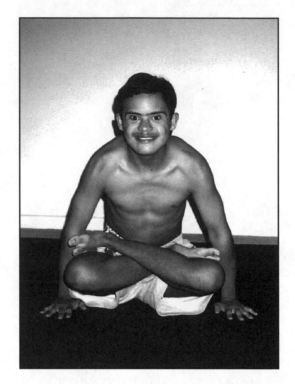

Henrique

Sonia Sumar was the first person to teach me to believe in my child. She taught me that the love I felt for him would surely help us to build a brighter future together.

I now see the birth of Henrique and the death of my older son, Elber, as the beginning of a new phase in my life. With Sonia's help, I have learned to give up my bitterness about the past. I have also learned to view the passing events of my life, tragic as well as joyous, with a measure of equal vision.

Maria de Lourdes Ramos de Souza
Belo Horizonte, March 14, 1994

Part Two

A Yoga Handbook
for the Special Child

3

A Yoga Primer

Yoga is a scientific system of physical and mental practices that originated in India more than 3,000 years ago. Its purpose is to help each one of us achieve our highest potential and to experience enduring health and happiness. With yoga, we can extend our healthy, productive years far beyond the accepted norm and, at the same time, improve the quality of our lives.

The branch of yoga that forms the main focus of my teaching work with both adults and children is called Hatha Yoga. Hatha Yoga begins by working with the body on a structural level, helping to align the vertebrae, increase flexibility, and strengthen muscles and tendons. At the same time, internal organs are toned and rejuvenated; the epidermal, digestive, lymphatic, cardiovascular, and pulmonary systems are purified of toxins and waste matter; the nervous and endocrine systems are balanced and toned; and the brain cells are nourished and stimulated. The end result is increased mental clarity, emotional stability, and a greater sense of overall well-being.

Because yoga works on so many different levels, it has great potential as an effective therapy for chronic diseases and conditions that do not respond well to conventional treatment methods. For this reason, children with Down Syndrome and other developmental disabilities who practice yoga often surprise their parents and teachers with their quick mastery of basic motor, communicative, and cognitive skills. The same yoga routine also helps children with learning disabilities develop greater concentration, balance, and composure in their daily lives. Everyone gains some level of benefit. The only requirements are proper instruction and regular practice.

While studying the methods presented in this book, it is important to remember that yoga is not just a slow-motion calisthenics workout or superficial exercise routine. Anyone who practices correctly soon begins to appreciate the depth and breadth of its benefits. For this reason, I always recommend that the parents of special students enroll in an adult yoga class; then they can experience the effects of yoga for themselves. After a number of lessons, they may experience some of the following benefits: the relaxation and softening of deep inner tensions and blockages, a sense of body-mind equilibrium, and a feeling of energetic buoyancy that can carry one right through the most difficult of days.

At our teaching center, I often remind my students not to strain or force themselves. Yoga is not a contest or a "quick fix." Like the proverbial story of the tortoise and the hare, yoga favors quiet, consistent application over theatrical displays and superficial accomplishments. It does not require that we transform ourselves overnight into something beyond our capacity. Yoga begins by accepting our limitations, whatever they may be, and working with this self-acceptance as a base. In our daily practice, we gradually learn to transcend our limitations, one by one, and in this way, real and lasting progress is possible.

A Five-Limbed Tree of Yoga

At our teaching center in Brazil, we employ the same basic yoga methods taught around the world since the system began. For my work with special children, I divide these methods into five areas of practice: (1) asanas, or body postures; (2) pranayama, or breathing exercises; (3) cleansing practices; (4) music and sound therapy; and (5) deep relaxation.

Asana literally means "posture" or "pose." According to an ancient and authoritative text,[1] an asana is "a particular posture of the body, which is both steady and comfortable." I prefer to call these postures "psycho-physical," since they form the basis of yoga's mind-body integration work. More than a hundred classical poses, with as many variations, can be subdivided into two categories: active and passive. Active poses tone specific muscle and nerve groups, benefit organs and endocrine glands, and activate brain cells. The passive poses are employed primarily in meditation, relaxation, and pranayama practices. The complete

---

[1] *The Yoga Sutras of Patanjali*

set of yoga asanas covers the entire human anatomy, quite literally from the top of the head to the tips of the toes. Regular practice helps to correct postural and systemic irregularities, and maintains the entire physiology in peak condition.

The greatest benefit from practicing asanas comes when we learn how to relax in a given pose. Contrary to what most of us have been taught, real relaxation results from a state of deep concentration, in which the mind is totally focused on a single object. During the practice of asanas, the object of concentration is the body. The student focuses his mind on the incoming and outgoing breaths, the steady flexion and extension of different muscle groups, or other bodily sensations. Ideally this inward focus should be maintained throughout the entire yoga class.

Pranayama is the science of proper breathing. Breath is the main source of nourishment for all the cells of the body. We can live without food for weeks, without water for days, but without oxygen for only a few minutes. The average person uses only about one-seventh of his total lung capacity. By learning how to increase this capacity with deep abdominal breathing, plus specific pranayama practices, we can increase the flow of vital energy to various organs in our bodies, build our immunity to disease, and overcome many physical ailments.

The way we breathe also has a profound effect on the nervous system. Our brain cells use three times more oxygen than other body cells. By regulating the breath and increasing oxygenation to brain cells, we help to strengthen and revitalize both the voluntary and autonomic nervous systems. When practiced consistently, pranayama also has a powerful stabilizing effect on the mind and emotions.

At the beginning of each yoga class, we employ several pranayama practices in order to prepare students for the asanas that follow. Pranayama and asanas work hand-in-hand to balance and integrate different physiological functions and to help dissolve emotional blocks and negative habit patterns that can obstruct the flow of vital energy within the body.

Purification (cleansing) practices include: a pranayama practice for eliminating excess phlegm and mucus from the respiratory system; an eye exercise; and a special technique for isolating and rolling the abdominal muscles. When properly performed, this last technique gives a powerful self-massage to the organs of the abdomen, resulting in improved digestion and relief from constipation.

Music and Sound Therapy use rhythm and melody, combined with hand movements and sound combinations, to develop concentration, breath coordination, communication and motor skills, as well as appreciation for the essentials of tone and harmony. In addition, studies have shown that the repetition of certain sound patterns can produce a calming and healing effect on the nervous system and psyche. The concept of sound therapy is as ancient and natural as the chirping of birds, the pitter-patter of a summer rainfall, or the internal rhythms of our own heartbeat and respiration. By combining sound therapy techniques with traditional yoga practices, such as chanting and intonation, it is possible to create an ideal learning environment for all levels of yoga practitioners.

Deep Relaxation is traditionally the conclusion and culmination of every yoga session. During ten to twenty minutes of complete silence and immobility, deep relaxation allows the body to absorb all the benefits of the previous asanas, pranayama, and cleansing practices.

When working with infants and toddlers, soft music is combined with massage of the feet and nape of the neck to help induce relaxation. For children and adults, deep relaxation begins as they lie down on their backs with palms up and legs spread one to two feet apart. Using soft background music and muted lighting, the instructor gently guides students through the relaxation process, encouraging the release of physical tension and mental stress by bringing the attention to various parts of the body. Visualization and meditation techniques are used in this part of the practice, as students direct their minds to points of tension and areas of blockage in their bodies. This is followed by a short period of unstructured relaxation. The session ends by bringing the students' awareness back to the body.

In life, it is necessary to learn how to relax after a period of activity. People spend approximately one third of their time in sleep, trying to recoup the energy and vitality they expended during the day. Unfortunately, many never achieve this objective because they have not learned the essentials of relaxation. Regular practice of deep relaxation helps to release tension and prevent the build-up of stress. As a result, our general level of health improves and our daily lives become more serene and harmonious.

4

The Early Stages of Development [1]

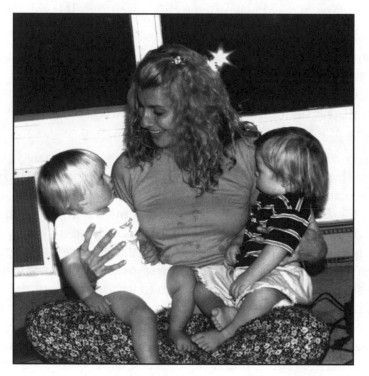

Over the years, as I continued to work with children who have special needs, I found it helpful to divide the progress of my students into several stages. This allowed me to create a specific program for each stage, tailoring the exercises and teaching methods to suit the various levels of the children's development.

Although I generally encourage parents to begin working with their child as soon as possible, there are instances when this is not advisable. Surgery or illness are valid reasons for postpone-

---

[1] For ease-of-use and clarity, I have chosen to alternate the gender of personal pronouns in the instruction section of this book. Chapter 4 uses the pronoun "he," Chapter 5 uses the pronoun "she," and so on.

ment. Sometimes parents do not hear about our program until their child is a teenager, and then they feel it is too late. This is a great mistake. Parents have enrolled their children at my teaching center from as early as two weeks to as late as fourteen years old; all of those who have continued with the program have had the satisfaction of witnessing great strides in their children's development.

Whatever the child's age, my first step is to evaluate the degree of developmental impairment so I can determine the appropriate program in which to place him. In some cases, there is a great disparity between the physical age and the developmental age of the child. In other cases, the child's motor and cognitive skills are much closer to the age-group average. No two children are exactly the same, and their development rates will reflect these differences.

In Chapters 5 through 8, I present a series of remedial programs designed for my yoga students with special needs. Each of these four chapters focuses on a different stage in the child's development. An outline of these stages and their specific areas of focus follows:

The Preparatory Stage (Birth to Six Months)[2]

The Preparatory Stage Program consists of a series of eleven exercises designed to prepare the infant or child for the practice of asanas. In this phase of development, the child is totally passive during the yoga session, absorbing the benefits of the exercises without any noticeable response.

The Inductive Stage (Six Months to One Year)

The Inductive Stage Program contains many of the same exercises as the Preparatory Stage, plus a number of basic asanas that are relatively easy to perform. As motor control and body awareness gradually develop, the child begins to respond by flexing or extending in accordance with the guiding movements of the instructor. Eventually the level of development reaches a point where the child is able to remain in a comfortable and steady pose for brief periods with the help of the instructor.

---

[2] "Birth to Six Months" refers to the developmental age of a child in the Preparatory Stage. For example, a six-year-old child with the motor development of a five-month-old baby will need to begin working in this stage.

The Interactive Stage (One to Two Years)

In the Interactive Stage Program, the child learns to participate in a greater variety of movements and poses. As the participation level increases, his need for assistance decreases. He will quickly learn to hold some of the poses without help, and others, with the touch of a hand. The instructor's task at this time is to provide him with just enough support to go into and hold a given pose without strain or discomfort.

The Imitative Stage (Two to Three Years)

In this stage, the child's motor and cognitive skills are developed enough to stand and walk without assistance, and to imitate the movements of others. Now it is time for him to start practicing asanas and pranayama with a minimum of physical assistance from the instructor. To facilitate this process, the parent or yoga instructor should be able to perform a basic yoga routine, since the child will learn most quickly by imitating others.

At our teaching center, classes for all four of the above stages are conducted on an individual basis. Children are encouraged to attend a minimum of two half-hour classes a week. Although the duration for each stage is listed as either six months or one year, these time frames can vary considerably. This depends on the child's age, capacity, and home environment, as well as the regularity of practice. Naturally, parents who are able to carry on with their child's yoga routine at home will see quicker and more far-reaching results.

The benefits of yoga therapy can be illustrated by a research project that was undertaken by my daughter Renata in 1994, as part of her thesis for a degree in Speech Pathology. This project consisted of personal interviews with the parents of eight of my yoga students at our center in Belo Horizonte. Each of these eight students has Down Syndrome. Two of them are boys, and the other six are girls. Their ages ranged from three to fourteen years, and all of them regularly attended two yoga classes per week. Several are still enrolled at my yoga school; others practiced yoga for a minimum of two to three years.

The interviews consisted of questions to the parents about their children's major developmental milestones in several key areas: gross motor skills, communication skills, and personal/social development. The results were compared with the development rates of two other groups of children: children without disabilities, and children with Down Syndrome who had never practiced yoga, but had received some other form of early intervention therapy[3] (refer to the table on the following page).

Several variables influenced the overall accuracy of this survey. First of all, some of the children who took part in my daughter's research project did not begin yoga therapy until they were more than a year old. Another variable was the number of times per week the parents conducted their children's practice sessions. Nevertheless, the yoga control group still outperformed the other Down Syndrome group in almost every area of development. In six of the milestone categories ("sits alone," "first word," "responsive smile," "finger-feeds," "bowel control," and "dresses oneself"), the yoga control group statistics were close to those of children without disabilities.

At our center, I always begin a course of yoga therapy with a personal evaluation of the prospective student and an interview with the parents. Normally, I ask parents to fill out a questionnaire that I have created for my yoga students with special needs (see questionnaire at the end of this chapter). To evaluate your child, you will first need to review your questionnaire, paying special attention to questions 15 through 20. Questions 15 through 20 deal with specific medical conditions that might contraindicate placing your child in certain yoga postures.

If your child is on medication, check with your pharmacist or pediatrician to make sure that it is safe to place him in an inverted position. If your child has seizures, suffers from a cardiac or spinal problem, or has had a recent illness or surgery, you will need to contact a yoga teacher who is certified to practice the methods outlined in this book.[4] The yoga teacher will be able to assess your child's needs and, in consultation with your physician, prepare a yoga program that your child can safely follow. *In such instances, do not attempt to begin a program of yoga therapy without professional guidance.*

The next step is to perform an evaluation of your child's motor skills and ability to respond to sensory stimuli.

---

[3] The development rates of children without disabilities and children with Down Syndrome, as well as other data pertaining to the table on page 62, were taken from a table on page 49 of *Down Syndrome: The Facts*, by Mark Selikowitz (Oxford University Press, 1990).

[4] A nationwide listing of yoga teachers certified in the Yoga for the Special Child™ teaching methods is available through our office at (804) 969-2668. A listing can also be found on the Yoga for the Special Child website at www.specialyoga.com.

Major Developmental Milestones

Areas of Development	Child without Disabilities		Yoga Control Group*		Child with Down Syndrome	
	Average age	Age range	Average age	Age range	Average age	Age range
I. Gross Motor Skills						
Sits alone	6 months	5–9 months	7 months	6–9 months	11 months	6–30 months
Crawls	9 months	6–12 months	14 months	11–24 months	15 months	8–22 months
Stands	11 months	8–17 months	19 months	10–30 months	20 months	12–39 months
Walks alone	14 months	9–18 months	22 months	16–36 months	26 months	12–48 months
II. Language Skills						
First word	12 months	8–23 months	15 months	10–24 months	23 months	12–48 months
Two-word phrases	2 years	15–32 months	3 years	1⅓–5 years	3 years	2–7½ years
III. Personal/Social Skills						
Responsive smile	1½ months	1–3 months	2 months	1–4 months	3 months	1½–5 months
Finger-feeds	10 months	7–14 months	11 months	7–18 months	18 months	10–24 months
Drinks from cup	13 months	9–17 months	18 months	9–24 months	23 months	12–32 months
Uses spoon	14 months	12–20 months	26 months	12–30 months	29 months	13–39 months
Bowel control	22 months	16–42 months	28 months	18–36 months	45 months	2–7 years
Dresses self	4 years	3¼–5 years	4½ years	3–7 years	7¼ years	3½–8¼ years

* Students with Down Syndrome at Sonia Sumar's yoga center

Motor Skills Evaluation

1. Check the child's ability to sit, stand, and walk. If you are a yoga teacher, educator, or health care professional, you can ask the parents a few simple questions before beginning the evaluation. Inquire about the child's basic motor skills, as well as any information in his questionnaire that may need clarification.
2. Remove the child's shoes. Check the formation of the feet, including arches, toes, and joints. Since the feet are the base for a good posture, healthy, well-formed feet will make it easier for him to stand and walk.
3. Put one of your fingers between each of the toes to check the child's grasping reflex in each foot, as well as the flexibility of the toes.
4. Check the degree of sensitivity in the feet by gently running your finger across the sole of each foot.
5. Check the alignment of the hips, legs and knees. Proper alignment of the lower limbs will affect the alignment of the spine and will also make it easier for the child to stand and walk.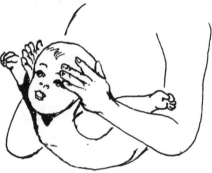
6. Check the formation of the chest, shoulders, arms, wrists, hands, and corresponding joints.
7. Check the grasping reflex in each hand.
8. Check the strength of the neck muscles in the following manner:

    I.   Place the child face down on a mat or blanket.
    II. Call to him. When you call, he will try to raise his head.
    III. If he cannot perform this movement, kneel down with your knees positioned on either side of the child's legs. Slide your arms forward under his upper arms and place your palms on either side of his head. Supporting his cheeks with your palms and the temples and forehead with your fingers, give him just enough help to raise his head off the floor.
    IV. If the child shows any signs of discomfort, immediately lower his head and turn him over onto his back.

    The child's ability to perform this muscle test will give you an indication of his physical strength, reflexes, and body awareness.

9. Bend the knees and elbows to check the mobility of the joints.
10. Hold the child in your arms in order to feel his muscle tone.

You will be able to assess the child's needs and choose a suitable yoga therapy program for him based on the following five factors: (1) muscle tone; (2) reflexes; (3) flexibility; (4) bone formation; and (5) structural alignment. You can also use the following guidelines in your evaluation:

Preparatory Stage Requirements

An infant or child who has not yet acquired any basic motor skills will need to begin with the Preparatory Stage Program. The absence of basic motor skills is indicative of early infancy, a nervous system dysfunction, or extremely low or high muscle tone. Children with Down Syndrome and cerebral palsy often need to begin working in this stage.

Inductive Stage Requirements

An infant or child who demonstrates some degree of body awareness and is able to participate minimally during the evaluation may begin with the Inductive Stage Program.

Interactive Stage Requirements

An infant or child who can sit alone and stand or walk with a minimum of assistance may begin with the Interactive Stage Program. In addition, he needs to have a basic understanding of your requests and commands. A child with attention deficit disorder, who has good motor skills but difficulty in following instructions, should begin working in this stage.

Imitative Stage Requirements

A child with good muscle tone and reflexes, who can follow your instructions, imitate your movements, and stand and walk without assistance, may begin with the Imitative Stage Program.

If you are a yoga teacher, educator, or health care professional, you can conduct your interview with the parents after completing the child's evaluation. Explain to them which program you have chosen as a starting point in your work with him. Take the time to discuss their home environment with them, focusing on their child's relationship with other family members. Ask them how they feel about his disability and what goals they expect him to achieve through yoga therapy. During this conversation it is important to uncover any hidden resentments or guilt that they might feel toward their child. Help them to understand the importance of learning to accept their child as he is. Acceptance will help them to develop a more positive and loving attitude toward their child, which will reinforce his self-confidence and encourage his development.

If you are a parent, the next step after evaluating your child is to determine a suitable yoga program for him. If you are unable to decide between two programs, choose the less advanced one. If he quickly masters the exercises in this routine, you can test him with several exercises from the more advanced program. Based on his response, you will know when he is ready to begin the next program.

As a parent, your responsibilities include creating a sup portive home environment, monitoring your child's diet, and conducting his yoga classes at home. I also encourage at least one parent to enroll in an adult yoga class. This helps to orient the parents to what their child is experiencing and to provide them with an appreciation of the techniques and benefits of yoga practice.

If you have the space, it is helpful to set aside a room in your house for the practice of yoga, where you can create a quiet and pleasant environment, free from interruptions. Your yoga room should be clean and have a comfortable floor covering, preferably carpeting. The decor should be simple and free of distracting objects, such as toys, magazines, books, television, etc. While other types of therapies may use toys and special equipment to stimulate your child's development, yoga uses breath, movement, physical posture, and the child's own voice to create an inward focus for developing concentration and body awareness. Therefore, the fewer "things" to distract him from this inner work, the better. The only exception to this general rule is a CD/cassette player, which I often use to drown out the noise of passing cars and other sounds from the outside. Religious hymns and chants can be especially conducive to the inward focus required for yoga practice, but a wide range of classical, new age, and ethnic music is also effective.

As a rule, I recommend that parents allow their child to wait at least two hours after eating or nursing before beginning a yoga session. Loose-fitting clothes are recommended so the child's movements are not restricted in any of the postures or breathing practices. For infants, a folded quilt, soft blanket, or fluffy towel can serve as a mat for yoga practice. Always have a change of diapers close by. For maximum benefit, try to follow the proper sequence in each of the yoga routines.

You and your child are now ready to take your first steps on the ancient path of yoga. Yoga stimulates all the areas necessary for an infant's development, so you should put your mind at ease and have faith in your child's innate capacity for growth and improvement. The best way to demonstrate this faith is by giving your baby lots of love and encouragement. This will help him to develop self-confidence and trust, qualities that will contribute to the success of this program.

Questionnaire for Parents of Yoga Students

Date:_____

1. Child's name_____

2. Date of birth_____Current age_____

3. Weight (at birth)_____ Length_____

4. Name and telephone number of child's pediatrician_____

   phone #_____

5. Comments on labor and delivery_____

6. Mother's name_____

7. Father's name_____

8. Brothers_____

9. Sisters_____

10. Have any family members practiced yoga?_____If so, how long?_____

11. What was the diagnosis of your child at birth?_____

2. What was the doctor's original prognosis for the future of your child?_____

   _____

13. What is the diagnosis of your child at present?_____

14. What are the physical symptoms of the disability?_____

15. Does your child have convulsions? (please describe)_____

16. Does your child have a cardiac problem? (please describe)_____

17. Does your child have a problem with his spinal column?_____In what area?

   _____

18. Has your child undergone surgery? (please describe, with dates)_____

_____

19. What medication does your child receive?_____

20. Can you think of any other reason, such as a recent physical illness or chronic

condition, that might contraindicate the practice of certain yoga poses?_____
_____

21. Briefly describe your child's dietary regimen._____

22. What other treatments or therapies has your child undergone? (please specify when and for how long)_____

23. Is your child's motor development delayed? (please describe)_____
_____

24. How would you describe your child's concentration, attention span, and general awareness?_____

25. Would you characterize your child as happy, aggressive, easygoing, enthusiastic, passive, excitable, depressed, introverted, or extroverted?_____
_____

26. How would you describe your child's relationship
    (a) with you?_____
    (b) with other family members? (be specific)_____
    (c) with friends?_____

27. Please describe the attitude of other family members toward your child (i.e., are they accepting, supportive, etc.)._____
_____

28. Do you have any evaluations by teachers, doctors, or therapists, including letters and reports? (Please attach copies when possible)_____

29. How did you hear about yoga therapy, and what goals do you hope your child will achieve by participating in this program?_____

5

The Preparatory Stage
Early Intervention
(Birth to Six Months)

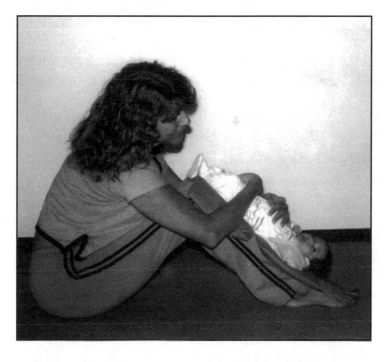

Within the first six months of life a child is generally most receptive to the long-term benefits of a remedial yoga program. At this time it is important for the yoga teacher to develop a strong, intuitive bond with his or her student. We refer to this process as "integration." The first yoga session with a new student is devoted exclusively to establishing channels of communication for this bonding process to take place.

With parents, bonding begins even before childbirth, since the mother is carrying the child in her womb. For mother and father, integration comes as a natural and positive development of loving their child. Therefore, it is often easier for them to achieve the degree of integration necessary for implementing a program of yoga therapy.

Before you begin working with your child, check your yoga classroom to make sure it has plenty of fresh air, but be careful to avoid drafts. Lights should be adjusted so they are not glaring (we often use blue or pink tinted bulbs because they give off a softer light). Many children respond positively to music and often prefer a particular style. A little experimentation with different cassettes will let you know which type of music to play for the best results. Remember to adjust the volume to a comfortable level that will not be distracting to the child.

The First Session

Begin the yoga session by placing your child face up on a folded blanket. Working on the floor, as opposed to a table or bed, is safer and allows both student and instructor more freedom of movement. Stay seated beside her at all times and try to avoid having other people enter the room during the session.

At this early stage, the sensory contact of massage is an excellent way to begin the work of bonding and integration. Sit at your child's feet and raise one of her legs several inches off the floor. With your free hand, wrap your fingers around the top of her raised foot, and place your thumb against the sole. Use your thumb in a gentle, kneading motion to massage the entire sole, working down from the toes to the heel. Be sure to include the inside arch of the foot. Then massage the top of the foot with your fingers. Repeat the same procedure with the other foot.

After the feet, slowly move up the body, massaging the legs, abdomen, arms, and so on, until you reach the top of the head. Talk to your baby while you work. Show the child that you really value this time together. Be gentle and affectionate. Little by little, you will achieve the empathy and integration necessary to create a climate of trust and harmony. Then you will be able to continue your work by gradually introducing a number of exercises that will prepare your child for the actual practice of yoga.

All Subsequent Sessions

☑ **Note:** Infants (and children who are not mobile) characteristically lack the muscular development of older, more active children. Their bone density is also relatively low. In the case of children with disabilities, the joints are sometimes prone to displacement. Therefore, the parent or professional who chooses to work with an infant must be careful not to force or strain the child's body in any of the following exercises. Start with the minimum duration or number of repetitions specified for each exercise. As your child becomes accustomed to the exercises, you will be able to gradually increase these limits. Allow short rest periods between exercises as necessary.

Exercises from a Supine[1] Position

Exercises for the Feet and Ankles

Benefits: These exercises promote strength and flexibility in the ankles and feet, help in the formation of the arches, and stimulate important energy points on the feet. The reason for starting with the feet is that they are the base for good posture when standing or walking. After performing these exercises, you may spend a few minutes massaging your child's feet. The relaxing effects of this massage will help to prepare her for the exercises that follow.

---

[1] Supine: lying on the back.

Exercise 1 | Foot Rotation

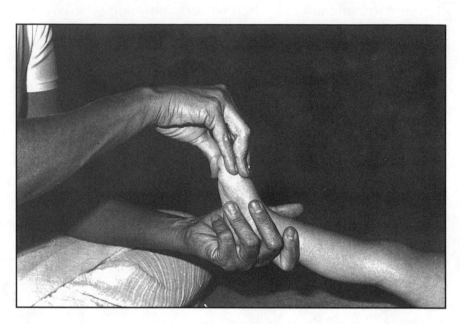

Technique:

1. Gently place your child on her back.

2. Take a comfortable seated position at her feet and place one of her heels in the palm of your upturned hand.

3. Wrap your fingers around the heel so that your thumb is pressing against one side of the ankle and your four fingers are pressing on the other side. This should secure the heel and immobilize the ankle joint.

4. With the other hand, hold the toes of the same foot and make circular movements with the upper part of the foot, first clockwise, then counterclockwise.

5. Do 2–4 repetitions in each direction and repeat with the other foot.

 Note: If your child's foot has a tendency to bend either inward or outward, the circular movement that puts pressure in the same direction will increase this tendency. If you emphasize movements in the opposite direction, the problem will be alleviated.

Ankle Flexion and Rotation | Exercise 2

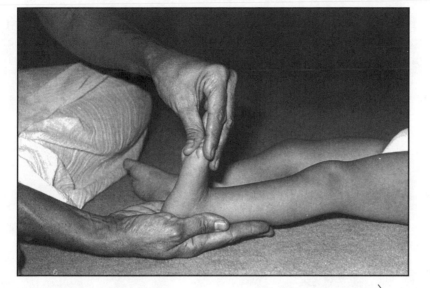

Technique:

1. Sit at your child's feet.

2. Hold one of her legs directly above the ankle.

3. Grasp the toes of the same foot with the tips of the fingers of your other hand.

4. Gently bend the toes and foot, first upward (away from you), then downward (toward you).

5. Do 2–4 repetitions.

6. Make circular movements with the toes, first clockwise, then counterclockwise.

7. Do 2–4 repetitions in each direction and repeat the entire exercise with the other foot.

☑ **Note:**

(1) If your child's foot has a tendency to bend either inward or outward, the circular movement that puts pressure in the same direction will increase this tendency. If you emphasize movements in the opposite direction, the problem will be alleviated.

(2) Follow Exercises 1 and 2 by massaging the soles of the feet. Use your thumbs in a kneading motion, working down from the toes to the heels of each foot. Be sure to include the inside arch of the foot.

Exercises for the Legs and Hips

Benefits: These exercises increase elasticity in the knees and hips, relieve tension in the lower back, and strengthen the tendons, nerves, and musculature of the legs. The exercises also have a stimulating effect on the organs of the abdomen and help to relieve gas, colic, and constipation.

Exercise
3

Supine Knee Bends

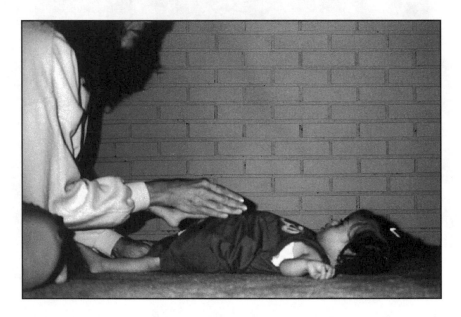

Technique:

1. Sit at your child's feet.

2. Place your left hand on top of her right thigh.

3. With your right hand, grasp her left leg directly below the knee.

4. Slowly raise the left leg off the floor, allowing the knee to flex at the same time. Use your left hand to help stabilize her body, making sure that the right leg remains flat on the floor.

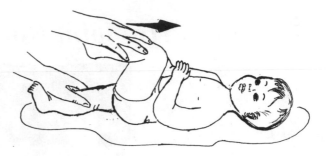

5. Push gently against the raised leg to increase the flexion in the knee. As you do so, the knee will pivot up over the hips, and the thigh will approach, or possibly even touch, the chest. Stop at the point where you feel resistance. Do not attempt to force the leg beyond this point.

6. Slowly return the right leg to its original position.

7. Do 1–2 repetitions and repeat with the other leg. Then perform the same exercise with both legs at the same time.

☑ **Note:**
(1) Make sure your child's body retains its alignment during all phases of this exercise by keeping both hips on the floor and the raised leg(s) from tilting either to the right or to the left.

(2) The goal of this exercise is to be able to touch your child's thigh to her chest; however, I have never seen a baby who was able to do this in the beginning. If you work slowly and patiently, the range of motion in the hip joint will gradually increase.

☒ **Caution:** If your child has had a colostomy, watch closely to make sure that she is not experiencing any discomfort. If necessary, reduce the degree of movement until you find an appropriate comfort level for performing this exercise.

Exercise 4 | *Hip Joint Rotation*

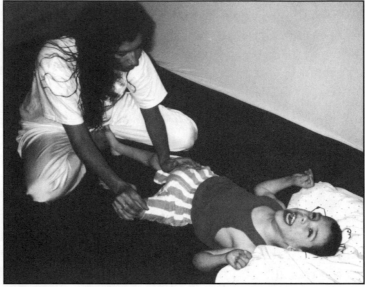

Technique:

1. Sit at your child's feet.

2. Place your right hand on top of her left thigh.

3. With your left hand, grasp her right leg directly below the knee.

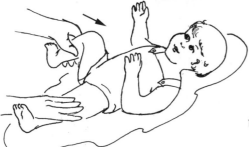

4. Raise the right leg with your left hand and gently swing it out to her right side as you flex the knee. Use your right hand to keep her left leg flat on the floor.

5. Moving the knee in an arc, guide it in toward the center of her chest.

6. Move the knee away from the chest in a straight line until the leg is fully extended. Viewed from above, you would see that her right knee had just completed a clockwise circle.

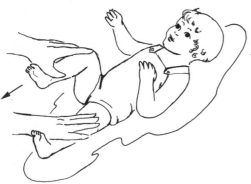

7. Do 2–4 repetitions and then perform the same exercise in a counterclockwise direction.

8. Repeat the clockwise and counterclockwise circles with the other leg. Then perform the same exercise with both legs at the same time.

☑ **Note:**
(1) Make sure your child's body retains its alignment during all phases of this exercise by keeping both hips on the floor.

(2) Remember not to force the legs. Always use the child's resistance as your guide.

☒ **Caution:** Remember to reduce the degree of movement and duration of the pose if your child has had a colostomy.

Exercises for the Torso

Supine Spinal Twist | *Exercise* 5

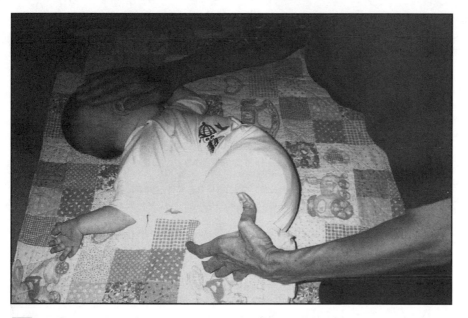

☒ **Caution:** Because the Supine Spinal Twist rotates the cervical vertebrae, it should not be performed by children with atlanto-axial instability.[2] This condition affects 10–20 percent of children with Down Syndrome. If your child has atlanto-axial instability, follow the instructions for the Supine Spinal Twist Variation described at the end of this exercise.

---

[2] Atlanto-axial instability is a condition of increased mobility in the joint between the atlas and the axis, the two cervical vertebrae at the base of the skull.

Benefits: The Spinal Twist is one of the most beneficial exercises for children with a nervous system dysfunction because it works the entire spinal column to keep it healthy and flexible. The twisting movements of the vertebrae stretch connecting ligaments, reduce disk compression, and stimulate nerves and ganglia in the area surrounding the spine. By compressing first one side of the body and then the other, this exercise massages and tones internal organs and glands, benefiting the liver, spleen, pancreas, kidneys, and adrenals. It also helps to relieve muscular tension in the back, waist, and hips.

Technique:

1. Sit at your child's feet.

2. Raise both legs together, bend her knees, and bring the thighs up toward the chest.

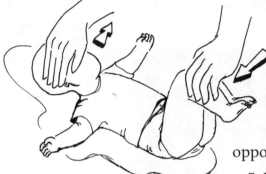

3. Grasp the knees with your left hand and place the palm of your right hand against her left cheek.

4. Slowly and gently rotate her head to the right, and her bent legs to the left. Her left knee should now be close to the floor or touching it, with the head turned in the opposite direction.

5. Hold this position for 3–6 seconds and return the head and bent legs to center.

6. Switch hands and repeat the Spinal Twist in the opposite direction.

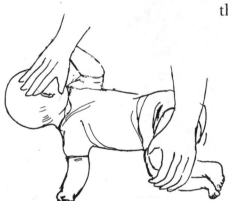

7. After completing the Spinal Twist in both directions, return both legs to the floor.

Note: The Supine Spinal Twist is a more advanced exercise and should not be performed during the first two months of yoga therapy. When you introduce this exercise, start with a 45-degree rotation in both directions and watch for any signs of discomfort. With each yoga session, you can increase the rotation by another 10–15 degrees, until you reach the child's limit.

Variation (for children with atlanto-axial instability):

1. Sit at your child's feet.

2. Raise both legs together, flex the knees, and bring the thighs in toward the chest.

3. Grasp the knees with your left hand and place the palm of your right hand on her right shoulder.

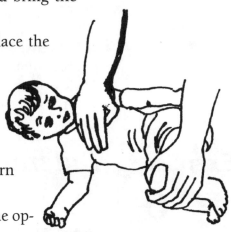

4. Slowly and gently rotate the bent legs to the left until the left knee is close to the floor or touching it. Press down on the right shoulder just enough to keep it from lifting off the floor.

5. Hold this position for 3–6 seconds and return the bent legs to center.

6. Switch hands and repeat the Spinal Twist in the opposite direction.

7. After completing the Spinal Twist in both directions, return both legs to the floor.

Exercises for the Arms and Upper Chest

Benefits: These exercises develop upper body strength, motor coordination, and lung capacity. Because the arm movements take place within the line of the child's vision, they also help to develop a sense of body awareness.

Exercise
6

Lateral Arm Raise

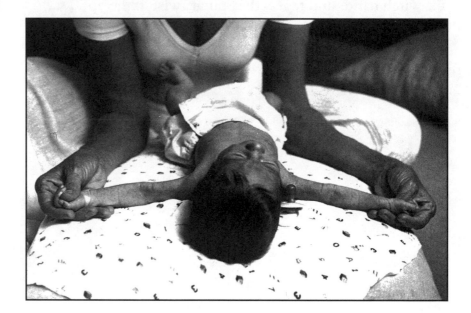

Technique:

1. Sit at your child's feet.

2. Stretch her arms out to each side so they form a straight line with the shoulders.

3. Turn her palms face up. Place your thumbs in the palms of her upturned hands and your fingers under the backs of her hands. The touch of your thumbs will stimulate a grasping response, and she will try to wrap her fingers around your thumbs.

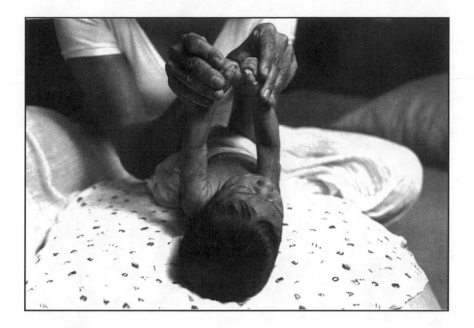

4. Raise her left arm and bring it to a vertical position above her chest.

5. Return the arm to the floor and stretch both arms by gently pulling them in opposite directions.

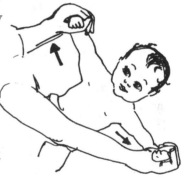

6. Do 2–4 repetitions and repeat with the other arm.

7. Perform the same exercise with both arms at the same time. Try to bring the two hands together when you raise them above the chest.

8. Raise the left arm, this time allowing it to bend at the elbow so that the upper arm remains on the floor.

9. Continue to bend the arm until you feel resistance, then return it to the floor.

10. Do 2–4 repetitions and repeat with the other arm.

☑ Note: As the grasping response gradually develops, your child will be able to hold your thumbs more firmly. The more firmly she grasps your thumbs, the less you will need to support her hands during this and the following exercise. Eventually she will be able to hold onto your thumbs throughout both exercises without any additional support.

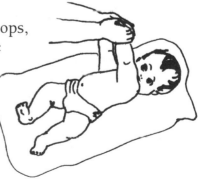

Exercise 7 | *Parallel Arm Raise*

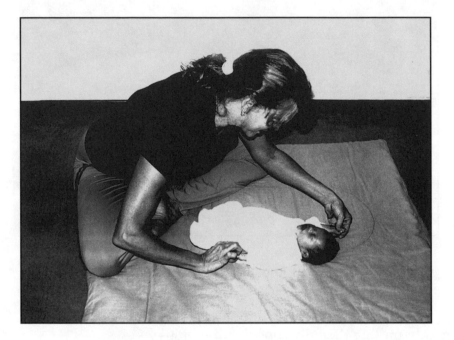

Technique:

1. Sit at your child's feet.

2. Place her arms alongside her body.

3. Put her palms face down. Place your thumbs in her palms and your fingers over the backs of her hands. The touch of your thumbs will stimulate a grasping response, and she will try to wrap her fingers around your thumbs.

4. Without bending her left arm, lift it straight up and over her head to the floor. Try to find the path of least resistance so that you are following the natural movement of her shoulder joint.

5. Stretch the arm as it reaches the floor beside her head.

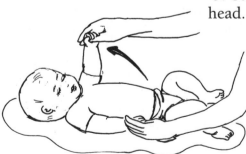

6. Reverse the movement and return the arm to its original position.

7. Do 2–4 repetitions and repeat with the other arm.

8. Perform the same exercise with both arms at the same time.

Exercises from a Prone[3] Position

Prone Leg Lifts | Exercise 8

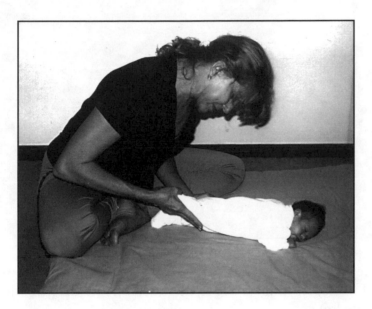

Benefits: This exercise strengthens the muscles of the lower back and buttocks, stretches the abdominal muscles, and tones the organs of the abdomen.

Technique:

1. Place your child face down, with her legs together.

2. Sit at her feet and place the palm of your left hand on her lower back.

3. With your right hand underneath her left knee, slowly raise her extended leg off the floor. Use your left hand to stabilize her body by keeping her left hip on the floor.

4. Stop at the point of resistance and slowly return the leg to the floor.

5. Do 2–4 repetitions and repeat with the other leg.

6. Perform the same exercise with both legs at the same time.

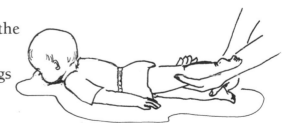

---

[3] Prone: Lying with the front or face downward.

Exercise 9 | *Prone Knee Bends*

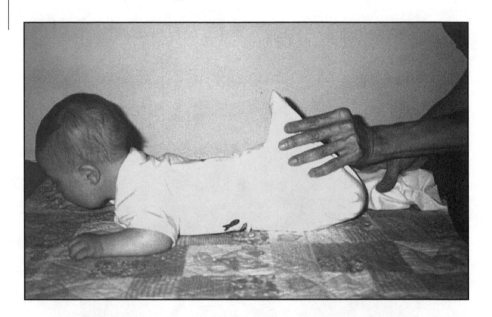

Benefits: Prone Knee Bends help to strengthen the musculature of the legs, elongate the thigh muscles, and increase flexibility in the knees.

Technique:

1. Sit at your child's feet.

2. Place your right hand on the calf of her right leg.

3. With your free hand, grasp her left leg just above the ankle and raise it off the floor, allowing the knee to flex as you bring the heel toward the buttocks.

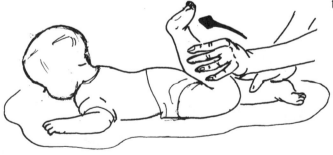

4. Stop at the point of resistance and lower the leg to the floor. Use your right hand to keep the child's right leg from lifting up.

5. Do 2–4 repetitions and repeat with the other leg.

6. Perform the same exercise with both legs at the same time.

Inverted Postures

Preparation for the Headstand

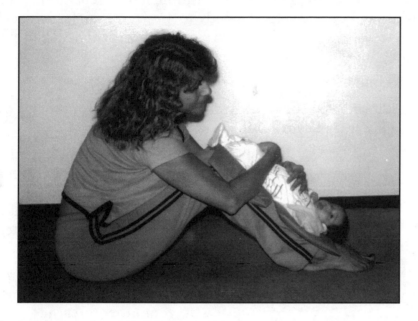

☒ **Caution:** If your child is on medication, check with your pharmacist or pediatrician to make sure that it is safe to place the child in an inverted position. If your child has a cardiac problem or seizures, then you should contact a yoga teacher who is certified to practice the methods outlined in this book. The yoga teacher will be able to assess your child's needs and, in consultation with your physician, prepare a yoga program that your child can safely follow.

Benefits: By reversing the pull of gravity, the Headstand redirects the flow of blood and lymph[4] throughout the entire body. Stagnant blood is drained from the legs, and the brain and upper endocrine glands are bathed in an increased supply of fresh, oxygen-rich blood. This pose benefits the entire nervous system, as well as the sense organs that are connected to the brain through the nerves. Scientific tests have shown that the Headstand improves memory and intellect.

---

[4] Lymph: a clear, yellowish fluid, containing white blood cells in a liquid resembling blood plasma, which is derived from the tissues of the body and conveyed to the blood stream by the lymphatic vessels.

This pose also aids digestion and elimination, alleviates urinary problems, tones internal organs, and reduces the risk of hernias and varicose veins. Because of these accumulated benefits, an overall sense of well-being is experienced by students who regularly practice this asana. In the yoga lexicon, the Headstand is known as the "King of Asanas." Although the Preparation for the Headstand only inverts the body to 45-degree angle, your child still receives many of the above-mentioned benefits from practicing this preparatory pose.

Technique:

1. Sit with your outstretched legs touching one another. Cover your lower legs with a thin cushion or folded towel.

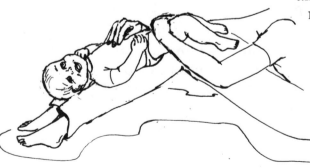

2. Place your child on top of the cushion in a supine position, so that her feet are resting on your thighs, and her head is resting just above your ankles. Make sure her spine is centered between your legs.

3. Secure her thighs with one of your forearms and her upper body with your other forearm.

4. Slowly raise your knees until your legs form an inverted "v." Be careful not to increase the incline of your legs to more than a 45-degree angle from the floor. You are now using your lower legs as a slantboard, with the child's head resting at the lowest point of the incline.

5. Begin by holding this pose for about ten seconds and gradually increase to a maximum of two minutes.

6. To come out of the pose, slowly lower your legs to the floor. Gently move your child to a blanket, without raising her head, and allow her to rest on her back.

Notes:

(1) Make sure your child's body does not slide down your legs as you go into and out of the pose.

(2) It is important to allow your child to rest on her back for at least one minute after performing the Preparation for the Headstand, so that the blood pressure can equalize throughout the body. If you raise her head too soon, it may cause her to become faint.

(3) Like the Spinal Twist, the Preparation for the Headstand is a more advanced exercise and should not be performed during the first two months of yoga therapy. After that, if there are no contraindications, then you can carefully introduce this exercise.

Conclusion to the Yoga Session

Exercise

11

Deep Relaxation

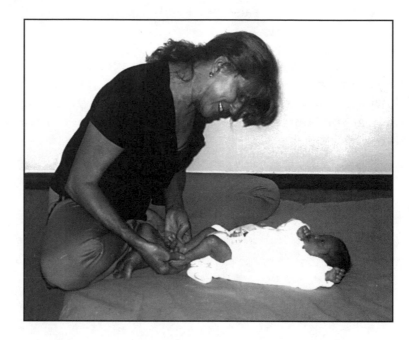

Benefits: Approximately 20 minutes have passed since the beginning of the yoga session, during which your child has had many areas of her body stretched and toned. Now it is time for her to rest, in order to assimilate the beneficial effects of all these movements and postures. In yoga, this is accomplished through Deep Relaxation. During Deep Relaxation, as muscles and nerves release stored-up tensions, a sense of calm and focus is restored. The nervous system is strengthened and general health improves. For this reason, I recommend that you always include Deep Relaxation as an integral part of your child's yoga routine.

Technique:

During Deep Relaxation your child should be kept as comfortable and still as possible. Try not to make any sudden movements that might distract her attention from the interior process that is taking place. If you wish to speak, do so quietly and in a soothing tone of voice.

Having just completed the Preparation for the Headstand, your child should now be resting on her back. Prepare the room by dimming the lights and putting on a cassette or CD of quiet, relaxing music. If the room seems cool or drafty, cover her with a blanket. Sit at her feet and place them 6–12 inches apart. Begin the relaxation process by massaging both feet at the same time. Massage the soles, using your thumbs in a gentle kneading motion. Then massage the top of each foot with your fingers. Allow her legs to remain resting on the floor while you massage her feet.

Depending on the child, you may wish to continue working on her feet throughout the entire relaxation period, or you may decide to stop massaging after a few minutes. Some children respond positively if you massage them from feet to head, naming each part of the body as you work on it. This type of verbal communication can help to develop greater body awareness. Other children prefer to be massaged on the nape of the neck, the face, or the top of the head. If the child has difficulty relaxing on the floor, you can try cradling her in your arms. Sometimes the closeness of this type of physical contact helps to induce a state of relaxation.

Feel free to structure the relaxation period according to your own perception of your child's needs. By being positive, intuitive, affectionate, and loving, you will find the best way to help her relax. Don't worry if she falls asleep — she will continue to absorb the benefits of Deep Relaxation. After approximately 10 minutes, bring your child out of Deep Relaxation by chanting or gently touching the soles of her feet. Finish the yoga session with some words of encouragement and (if you wish) several hugs and kisses.

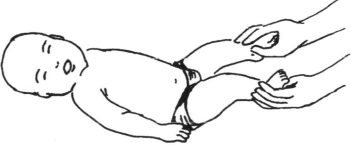

Notes and Comments on the Preparatory Stage

- A complete yoga session, including Deep Relaxation, should last no longer than 30 minutes.

- Be consistent. A little yoga every day will be much more effective in the long run than a lot of yoga once in a while.

- Remember to allow time in between exercises for your child to relax in preparation for the next exercise.

- If your child's motor development is severely impaired, she will need professional help. Contact a yoga teacher who is certified to practice the methods outlined in this book. The yoga teacher will be able to assess your child's needs and prepare a yoga program adapted to the level of your child's development.

- **If your child has seizures, suffers from a cardiac or spinal problem, or has had a recent illness or surgery, do not attempt to begin a program of yoga therapy without professional guidance.** You will need to contact a yoga teacher who is certified to practice the methods outlined in this book. The yoga teacher will be able to assess your child's needs and, in consultation with your physician, prepare a yoga program that your child can safely follow.

- Developing speech and language skills requires the assistance of a speech and/or language therapist. Yoga helps to improve respiration and will complement the work of the therapist.

- Keep in mind that it can take up to a month for teacher and child to achieve the level of integration necessary for productive yoga therapy sessions. Sometimes the "chemistry" between teacher and student makes bonding difficult. If you continue to experience resistance after the initial month, it may be best to look for another yoga teacher, hopefully one with whom the child feels a greater rapport.

Yoga Practice Charts for the Preparatory Stage

Once you have become familiar with the Preparatory Stage exercises, you may use the easy-reference chart on the following page to guide you through your child's yoga routine. Some parents also find it helpful to keep a daily record of their child's yoga practice. Following the easy-reference chart is a weekly yoga chart that you may use for this purpose.

Preparatory Stage Exercises

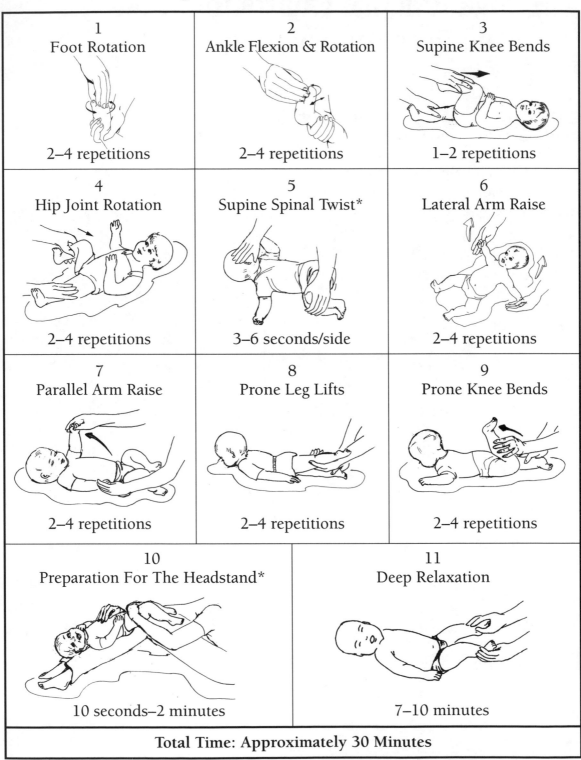

1 Foot Rotation 2–4 repetitions	**2** Ankle Flexion & Rotation 2–4 repetitions	**3** Supine Knee Bends 1–2 repetitions
4 Hip Joint Rotation 2–4 repetitions	**5** Supine Spinal Twist* 3–6 seconds/side	**6** Lateral Arm Raise 2–4 repetitions
7 Parallel Arm Raise 2–4 repetitions	**8** Prone Leg Lifts 2–4 repetitions	**9** Prone Knee Bends 2–4 repetitions
10 Preparation For The Headstand* 10 seconds–2 minutes		**11** Deep Relaxation 7–10 minutes

Total Time: Approximately 30 Minutes

* The Spinal Twist and Preparation for the Headstand are more advanced exercises and should not be performed during the first two months of yoga therapy.

Monthly Yoga Chart

Student's Name:

Month:

Year:

Starting Date:

	1	2	3	4	5	6	7	8	9	10	11	12	13	14	15	16	17	18	19	20	21	22	23	24	25	26	27	28	29	30	31
1) Foot Rotation																															
2) Ankle Flexion & Rotation																															
3) Supine Knee Bends																															
4) Hip Joint Rotation																															
5) Supine Spinal Twist																															
6) Lateral Arm Raise																															
7) Parallel Arm Raise																															
8) Prone Leg Lifts																															
9) Prone Knee Bends																															
10) Preparation for Headstand																															
11) Deep Relaxation																															

Remarks:

6

The Inductive Stage
Initiating Asanas
(Six Months to One Year)

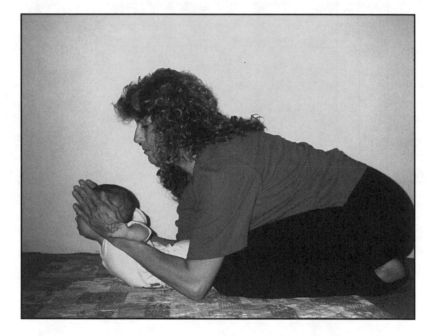

After your child has been practicing yoga for a number of months, you will start to observe subtle changes in the way he is able to perform the Preparatory Stage exercises. He will seem more relaxed during his yoga sessions. You will notice that he is more conscious of his relationship with you and of the movements that you are performing with his body. You will perceive that he has more endurance and no longer needs rest periods between many of the exercises, even though you may have increased the number of repetitions. These are signs that your child has reached a transition period in his development and is ready to begin learning asanas in the Inductive Stage Program.

Of course, this description may not necessarily correspond to your own child's development. Even if you are unable to perceive any of above changes in your child, the benefits of yoga therapy are still accruing; it will just take a little longer before he is ready to advance to the next stage. Also, it is important to understand that there is no clear-cut line between the Preparatory and Inductive Stage Programs since both include many of the same exercises.

In order to begin working in the Inductive Stage Program, your integration with your child must be so complete that you can sense his changing moods, as well as his capacity to perform the various exercises that are part of his routine. Once you feel you have achieved this degree of integration, you can begin introducing the Inductive Stage exercises one at a time, carefully noting his reaction to each new exercise or pose.

As you continue to work with your child in this manner, he will gradually gain the necessary confidence and skill to accompany your guiding movements into and out of each pose. Thus, when being placed in a certain posture, he will not remain completely passive, but will collaborate by flexing or extending the appropriate muscle groups. At first, these synchronistic movements can be very subtle, so you must be attentive and "tuned in" to the child's body in order to sense these changes.

You may also notice a change in your child's respiratory pattern. During the exercises, his lungs will instinctively fill as his body moves upward, and empty as his body moves downward. This type of rhythmical breathing will help to expand his lung capacity and improve circulation. Also, by learning how to coordinate the breath and body movements, he will gradually gain control of his respiration, a prerequisite for practicing pranayama later on.

Over a period of months, as your child becomes more competent in his yoga practice, you can gradually extend the duration of individual poses and increase the degree of flexion, extension, or rotation. If you stay focused and aware, you will be able to sense the proper duration for each pose. Bring your child out of a pose a soon as his body sends you a signal that it has held the pose long enough. As your child's participation, self-confidence, and motor control continue to improve, his ability to remain in a steady and comfortable pose will also improve. Not until he is steady and comfortable in a particular pose does it become an asana in the classic sense of the word.

Note: Infants (and children who are not mobile) characteristically lack the muscular development of older, more active children. Their bone density is also relatively low. In the case of children with disabilities, the joints are sometimes prone to displacement. Therefore, the parent or professional who chooses to work with an infant must be careful not to force or strain the child's body in any of the following exercises. Start with the minimum duration or number of repetitions specified for each exercise. As your child becomes accustomed to the exercises, you will be able to gradually increase these limits. Allow short rest periods between exercises as necessary.

Exercises from a Supine[1] Position

Exercises for the Feet and Ankles

Benefits: Since one of the main objectives of Preparatory Stage Exercises 1–4 is to help prepare your child to walk, they are also included in this routine. These exercises promote strength and flexibility in the ankles and feet, help in the formation of the arches, and stimulate important energy points on the feet. The reason for starting with the feet is that they are the base for a good posture when standing or walking. After performing these exercises, you may spend a few minutes massaging your child's feet. The relaxing effects of this massage will help to prepare him for the exercises that follow.

---

[1] Supine: lying on the back.

Foot Rotation | *Exercise* 1

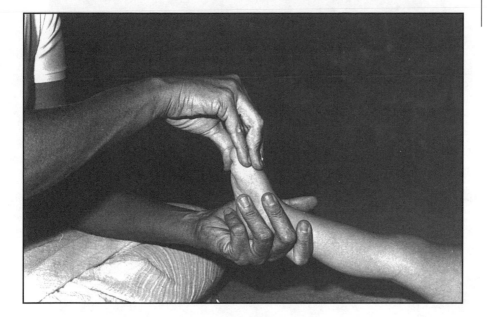

Technique:

1. Gently place your child on his back.

2. Take a comfortable seated position at his feet and place one of his heels in the palm of your upturned hand.

3. Wrap your fingers around the heel so that your thumb is pressing against one side of the ankle and your four fingers are pressing on the other side. This should secure the heel and immobilize the ankle joint.

4. With the other hand, hold the toes of the same foot and make circular movements with the upper part of the foot, first clockwise, then counterclockwise.

5. Do 2–4 repetitions in each direction and repeat with the other foot.

☑ **Note:** If your child's foot has a tendency to bend either inward or outward, any movement that puts pressure in the same direction will increase this tendency. If you emphasize movements in the opposite direction, the problem will be alleviated.

Exercise 2 | *Ankle Flexion and Rotation*

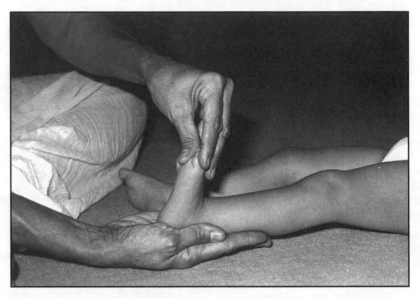

Technique:

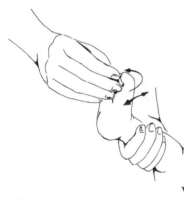

1. Sit at your child's feet.

2. Hold one of his legs directly above the ankle.

3. Grasp the toes of the same foot with the tips of the fingers of your other hand.

4. Gently bend the toes and foot, first upward (away from you), then downward (toward you).

5. Do 2–4 repetitions.

6. Make circular movements with the toes, first clockwise, then counterclockwise.

7. Do 2–4 repetitions in each direction and repeat the entire exercise with the other foot.

 Note:

(1) If your child's foot has a tendency to bend either inward or outward, any movement that puts pressure in the same direction will increase this tendency. If you emphasize movements in the opposite direction, the problem will be alleviated.

(2) Follow Exercises 1 and 2 by massaging the soles of the feet. Use your thumbs in a kneading motion, working down from the toes to the heels of each foot. Be sure to include the inside arch of the foot.

Exercises for the Legs and Hips

Benefits: These exercises increase flexibility in the knees and hips, relieve tension in the lower back, and fortify the tendons, nerves, and musculature of the legs. The exercises also have a stimulating effect on the organs of the abdomen and help to relieve gas, colic, and constipation.

Supine Knee Bends | *Exercise* 3

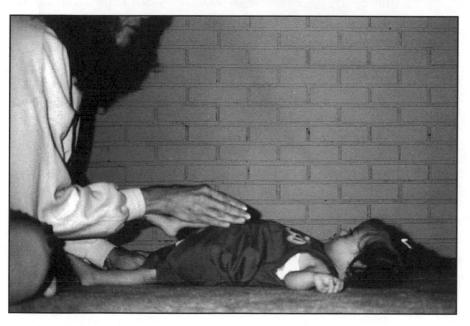

Technique:

1. Sit at your child's feet.

2. Place your left hand on top of his right thigh.

3. With your right hand, grasp his left leg directly below the knee.

4. Slowly raise the left leg off the floor, allowing the knee to flex at the same time. Use your left hand to help stabilize his body, making sure that the right leg remains flat on the floor.

5. Push gently against the raised leg to increase the flexion in the knee. As you do so, the knee will pivot up over the hips, and

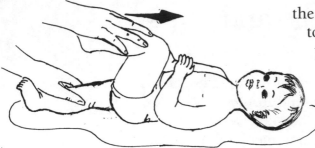

the thigh will approach, or possibly even touch, the chest. Stop at the point where you feel resistance. Do not attempt to force the leg beyond this point.

6. Slowly return the right leg to its original position.

7. Do 1–2 repetitions and repeat with the other leg. Then perform the same exercise with both legs at the same time.

 Note:

(1) Make sure your child's body retains its alignment during all phases of this exercise by keeping both hips on the floor and the raised leg(s) from tilting either to the right or to the left.

(2) The goal of this exercise is to be able to touch your child's thigh to his chest; however, I have never seen a baby who was able to do this in the beginning. If you work slowly and patiently, the range of motion in the hip joint will gradually increase.

 Caution: If your child has had a colostomy, watch closely to make sure that he is not experiencing any discomfort. If necessary, reduce the degree of movement until you find an appropriate comfort level for performing this exercise.

Hip Joint Rotation | Exercise 4

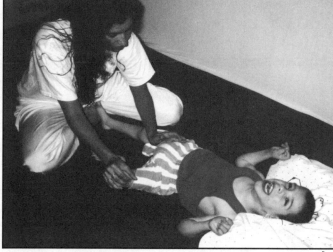

Technique:

1. Sit at your child's feet.

2. Place your right hand on top of his left thigh.

3. With your left hand, grasp his right leg directly below the knee.

4. Raise the right leg with your left hand and gently swing it out to his right side as you flex the knee. Use your right hand to keep his left leg flat on the floor.

5. Moving the knee in an arc, guide it in toward the center of his chest.

6. Move the knee away from the chest in a straight line until the leg is fully extended. Viewed from above, you would see that his right knee had just completed a clockwise circle.

7. Do 2–4 repetitions and then perform the same exercise in a counterclockwise direction.

8. Repeat the clockwise and counterclockwise circles with the other leg. Then perform the same exercise with both legs at the same time.

✔ **Note:** (1) Make sure your child's body retains its alignment during all phases of this exercise by keeping both hips on the floor. (2) Remember not to force the legs. Always use the child's resistance as your guide.

 Caution: Remember to reduce the degree of movement and duration of the pose if your child has had a colostomy.

Exercises for Strengthening the Muscles of the Abdomen

Exercise 5 | *Leg Lifts*

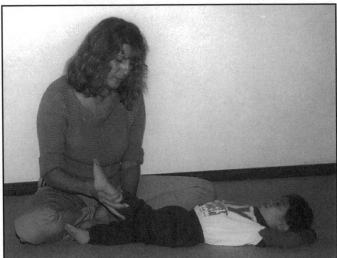

Benefits: This exercise strengthens the muscles of the abdomen and thighs. It also elongates the hamstrings and posterior muscles of the legs.

Technique:

1. Sit at your child's feet.

2. With your right hand, reach around to the outside of his left leg and grasp the left knee. The fingers of your right hand should now be resting on top of his left knee, with your thumb extending beneath the calf of his leg.

3. Using your thumb and fingers to keep his leg straight, raise it off the floor until it is vertical. Keep the other leg on the floor with your left hand.

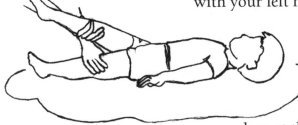

4. Hold this position momentarily, then return the right leg to the floor.

5. Do 2–4 repetitions and repeat with the other leg.

6. Perform the same exercise with both legs at the same time.

☑ **Note:** Make sure both of the child's hips remain on the floor during all phases of this exercise.

Exercises for the Torso

The Knee-to-Chest Pose

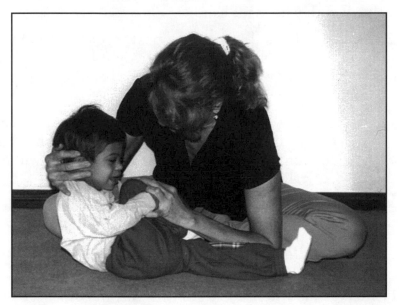

Benefits: Similar in appearance to Exercise 3, this pose is excellent for relieving gas, colic, and other intestinal problems. It strengthens the muscles of the abdomen, stretches the muscles of the back and neck, and helps to increase flexibility in the hips and knees. It is especially beneficial for relieving stress in the lower back.

Technique:

1. Sit to the left side of your child.

2. Place your right hand on top of his left thigh. Place your left hand on top of his right leg directly below the knee.

3. Grasp the right leg and raise it off the floor, allowing the knee to flex at the same time. Push gently against the leg to increase the flexion in the knee.

4. Replace your left hand with your right hand and lower your right forearm until it rests on top of his left leg. During the remainder of this exercise, you can use your right forearm to keep the left leg from lifting off the floor.

5. With your right hand, continue to push gently against the child's right leg. As you do so, the knee will pivot up over the

hips, and the thigh will approach, or possibly even touch, the chest.

6. Grasp his right hand with your left hand and place it on top of the bent knee. Keep his hand positioned on top of the knee by securing it with your right hand.

7. Grasp his left hand and place it next to, or overlapping, his right hand. Secure his hands with your right hand. Both of his hands should now be wrapped around the bent knee, as if they were pulling it in toward the chest.

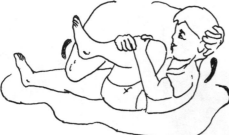

8. With your left hand, reach under the back of his head and raise it up. Try to touch the chin or forehead to the knee. As you do so, he will naturally exhale.

9. Hold this position until you feel him begin to inhale (about 2–4 seconds).

10. To help him come out of the pose, lower the head first, then the arms and leg to the floor.

11. Repeat the Knee-to-Chest Pose with the other leg. Then perform the same pose with both legs at the same time.

 Note: Make sure your child's body retains its alignment during all phases of this exercise by keeping both hips on the floor and the raised leg(s) from tilting either to the right or to the left.

 Caution: Remember to reduce the degree of movement and duration of the pose if your child has had a colostomy.

The Yogic Sleep Pose | Exercise 7

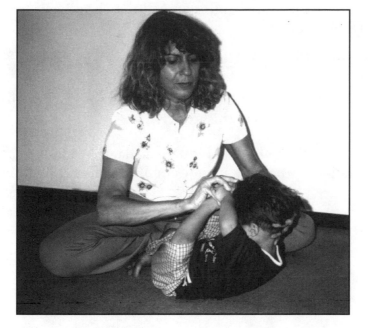

Benefits: This pose creates a forward-bending stretch along the entire spine. It also tones the organs of the abdomen and helps to increase flexibility in the hips and knees.

Technique:

1. Sit along the right side of your child.

2. Grasp both ankles and raise his legs off the floor until they are vertical.

3. With one hand on each ankle, separate the ankles and bring the soles of the feet together above the child's body. In order to accomplish this, you will need to lower both feet toward the chest, allowing the knees to bend outward in opposite directions.

4. Clasp the feet together with your right hand and use your left hand to bring his hands, one at a time, up to the feet. At this point, you should be holding his hands and feet together with your right hand.

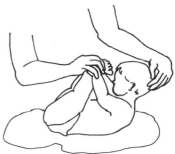

5. Reach under the back of his neck with your left hand and raise it up until the forehead touches the feet. The hands, feet, and forehead should ideally meet at a single point.

6. Hold this position until you feel the child begin to inhale (about 3–6 seconds).

7. To help him come out of the pose, lower the head first, then the arms and legs to the floor.

 Note: Make sure both of your child's hips remain on the floor during all phases of this exercise.

 Caution: Remember to reduce the degree of movement and duration of the pose if your child has had a colostomy.

Supine Spinal Twist | Exercise

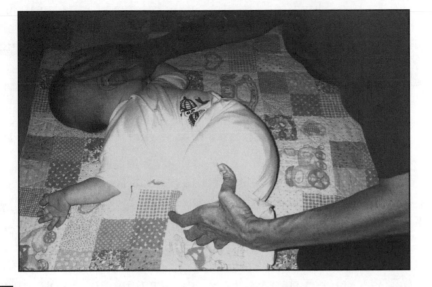

☒ Caution: Because the Supine Spinal Twist rotates the cervical vertebrae, it should not be performed by children with atlanto-axial instability.[2] This condition affects 10–20 percent of children with Down Syndrome. If your child has atlanto-axial instability, follow the instructions for the Supine Spinal Twist Variation described at the end of this exercise.

Benefits: The Spinal Twist is one of the most beneficial exercises for children with a nervous system dysfunction because it works the entire spinal column to keep it healthy and flexible. The twisting movements of the vertebrae stretch connecting ligaments, reduce disk compression, stimulate nerves and ganglia in the area surrounding the spine. By compressing first one side of the body and then the other, this exercise massages and tones internal organs and glands, benefiting the liver, spleen, pancreas, kidneys, and adrenals. It also helps to relieve muscular tension in the back, waist, and hips.

Technique:

1. Sit at your child's feet.

2. Raise both legs together, bend his knees, and bring the thighs up toward the chest.

---

[2] Atlanto-axial instability is a condition of increased mobility in the joint between the atlas and the axis, the two cervical vertebrae at the base of the skull.

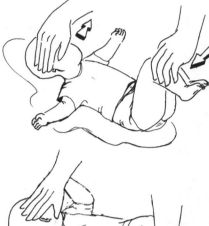

3. Grasp the knees with your left hand and place the palm of your right hand against his left cheek.

4. Slowly and gently rotate his head to the right, and his bent legs to the left. His left knee should now be close to the floor or touching it, with the head turned in the opposite direction.

5. Hold this position for 3–6 seconds and return the head and bent legs to center.

6. Switch hands and repeat the Spinal Twist in the opposite direction.

7. After completing the Spinal Twist in both directions, return both legs to the floor.

Note: The Supine Spinal Twist is a more advanced exercise and should not be performed during the first two months of yoga therapy. When you introduce this exercise, start with a 45-degree rotation in both directions and watch for any signs of discomfort. With each yoga session, you can increase the rotation by another 10–15 degrees, until you reach the child's limit.

Variation (for Children with Atlanto-Axial Instability):

1. Sit at your child's feet.

2. Raise both legs together, flex the knees, and bring the thighs in toward the chest.

3. Grasp the knees with your left hand and place the palm of your right hand on his right shoulder.

4. Slowly and gently rotate the bent legs to the left until the left knee is close to the floor or touching it. Press down on the right shoulder just enough to keep it from lifting off the floor.

5. Hold this position for 3–6 seconds and return the bent legs to center.

6. Switch hands and repeat the Spinal Twist in the opposite direction.

7. After completing the Spinal Twist in both directions, return both legs to the floor.

Exercises for the Arms and Upper Chest

Benefits: These exercises develop upper body strength, motor coordination, and lung capacity. Because the arm movements take place within the line of the child's vision, they also help to develop a sense of body awareness.

Lateral Arm Raise | Exercise 9

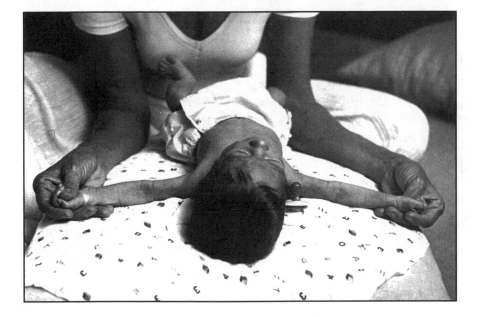

Technique:

1. Sit at your child's feet.

2. Stretch his arms out to each side so they form a straight line with the shoulders.

3. Turn his palms face up. Place your thumbs in the palms of his upturned hands and your fingers under the backs of his hands. The touch of your thumbs will stimulate a grasping response, and he will try to wrap his fingers around your thumbs.

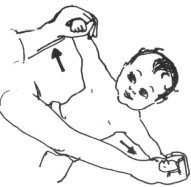

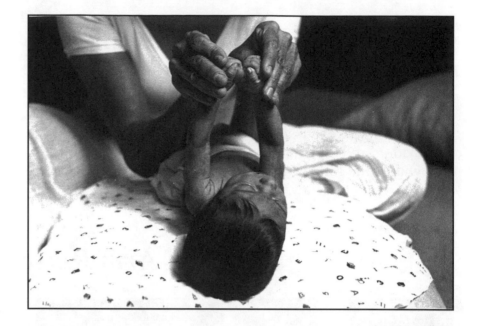

4. Raise his left arm and bring it to a vertical position above his chest.

5. Return the arm to the floor and stretch both arms by gently pulling them in opposite directions.

6. Do 2–4 repetitions and repeat with the other arm.

7. Perform the same exercise with both arms at the same time. Try to bring the two hands together when you raise them above the chest.

8. Raise the left arm, this time allowing it to bend at the elbow so that the upper arm remains on the floor.

9. Continue to bend the arm until you feel resistance, then return it to the floor.

10. Do 2–4 repetitions and repeat with the other arm.

☑ Note: As the grasping response gradually develops, your child will be able to hold your thumbs more firmly. The more firmly he grasps your thumbs, the less you will need to support his hands during this and the following exercise. Eventually he will be able to hold onto your thumbs throughout both exercises without any additional support.

Parallel Arm Raise | Exercise *10*

Technique:

1. Sit at your child's feet.

2. Place his arms alongside his body.

3. Put his palms face down. Place your thumbs in his palms and your fingers over the backs of his hands. The touch of your thumbs will stimulate a grasping response, and he will try to wrap his fingers around your thumbs.

4. Without bending his left arm, lift it straight up and over his head to the floor. Try to find the path of least resistance so that you are following the natural movement of his shoulder joint.

5. Stretch the arm as it reaches the floor beside his head.

6. Reverse the movement and return the arm to its original position.

7. Do 2–4 repetitions and repeat with the other arm.

8. Perform the same exercise with both arms at the same time.

Exercises from a Prone[3] Position
Backward-Bending Poses

Backward-bending poses form one of the four basic groups of asanas for the spine. The other three groups are forward-bending, twisting, and side-bending poses. The backward-bending poses reverse the stretch of the forward-bending poses; a left twist reverses the stretch of a right twist, and so on. Taken together, all four groups constitute a total program for keeping the spinal column flexible, healthy, and resilient. These complementary poses fortify the central nervous system, strengthen and elongate all the muscles of the torso, and benefit all the internal organs.

Exercise

11

The Cobra Pose

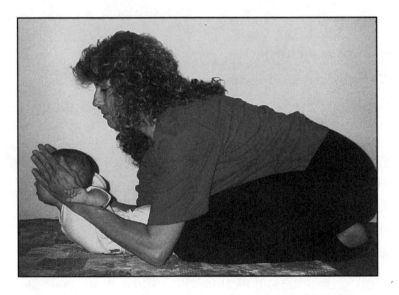

Benefits: This asana elongates the body's anterior muscles and helps to release tension from the solar plexus and lower back. It expands the rib cage, tones the heart, lungs, and cranial nerves, and strengthens the upper back and neck muscles. It also helps to correct spinal displacement and to relieve constipation and gas.

---

[3] Prone: lying with the front or face downward.

Technique:

1. Place your child face down.

2. Kneel down with your knees positioned on either side of the child's legs.

3. Slide your arms forward under his upper arms and place the palms of your hands against his cheeks. Support his temples and forehead with your fingers. Center the head so that it is twisting neither to the left nor to the right.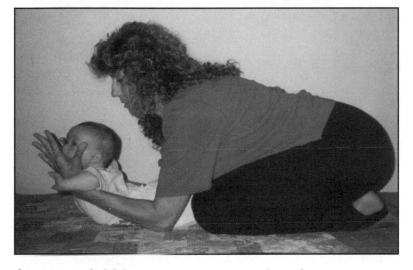

4. Using your elbows as pivots and your forearms as levers, gently raise his head and upper torso off the floor. As you lift, his head will come up first, then the neck and shoulders, and finally the chest.

5. Stop at the point of resistance and hold for 4–10 seconds.

6. To help him come out of the pose, slowly lower his head and upper torso to the floor in reverse order, beginning with the chest and ending with the head.

Advanced Variation:

After your child becomes accustomed to this asana, you can train his neck muscles by reducing the support of your hands while he is holding the pose. Slowly lower your hands, at the same time encouraging him to keep his head in an upright position. If he is unable to keep his head upright, then return your hands to their previous position. Continue experimenting over a period of weeks and months, and eventually he will be able to keep his head up without any support from your hands.

The Locust Pose

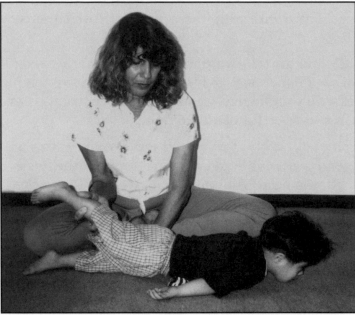

Benefits: This asana strengthens the muscles of the lower back and buttocks, stretches the abdominal muscles, and tones the organs and glands of the abdomen.

Technique:

1. Sit to the left side of your child.

2. Bring his legs together and position his arms alongside his body.

3. Place the palm of your left hand on his lower back.

4. With your right hand underneath his left knee, slowly raise his extended leg off the floor. Use your left hand to keep his left hip on the floor.

5. Stop at the point of resistance and hold the pose for 3–6 seconds.

6. To help him come out of the pose, slowly lower his leg to the floor.

7. Repeat the Locust Pose with the other leg. Then perform the same exercise with both legs at the same time.

The Half-Bow Pose | Exercise 13

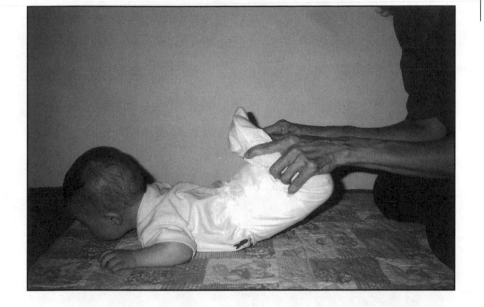

Benefits: This asana elongates the thigh muscles and provides many of the same benefits as both the Cobra and Locust Poses.

Technique:

1. Sit at your child's feet.

2. Grasp both legs just above the ankles.

3. Raise the legs off the floor, allowing the knees to bend at the same time.

4. Continue to bend the legs at the knees until the soles of the feet are facing the back of his head. At this point, his knees and thighs should be off the floor.

5. Hold the pose for 3–6 seconds.

6. To help him come out of the pose, slowly return the legs to the floor.

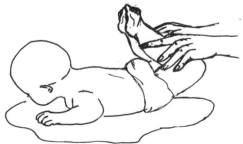

The Child Pose

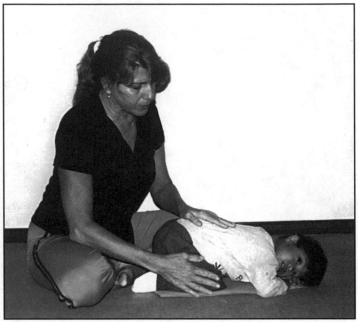

Benefits: Although technically not a backward-bending asana, the Child Pose is included in this section because it makes an excellent counter-pose to the previous three exercises. This asana creates a gentle forward-bending stretch that helps to elongate the spine and reduce disk compression, especially in the lower back. Like the Knee-to-Chest Pose, it helps to relieve colic, gas, and other intestinal problems.

Technique:

1. Sit at your child's feet.

2. Place one hand over both of his calves and the other hand (palm up) beneath his chest.

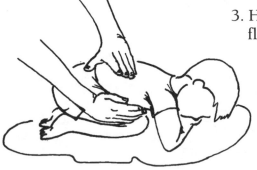

3. Hold the calves down and raise the chest off the floor.

4. Use your upturned hand to move his chest back toward his feet. As you do this, his knees will bend, and his hips will pivot up over the knees and down toward the floor. Continue the movement until his buttocks are resting on his heels.

5. Lower his chest onto his thighs. Remove your hands, and adjust both feet so that the soles are facing upward.

6. Help him maintain this position by placing one of your hands on his lower back and exerting a gentle downward pressure.

7. Hold this posture until you feel him trying to extend his legs (10–30 seconds).

8. To help him come out of the pose, place one hand over his calves and the other beneath his chest. Then return his upper body to a prone position.

☑ Note: During this exercise, be careful not to raise the child's chest so high that his head lifts off the floor. This will help to prevent neck strain.

Inverted Poses

Exercise
15

The Headstand

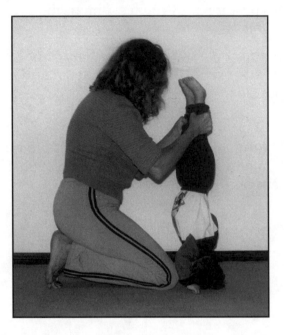

> ☒ **Caution:** If your child is on medication, check with your pharmacist or pediatrician to make sure that it is safe to place the child in an inverted position. If your child has a cardiac problem or seizures, then you should contact a yoga teacher who is certified to practice the methods outlined in this book. The yoga teacher will be able to assess your child's needs and, in consultation with your physician, prepare a yoga program that your child can safely follow.

Benefits: By reversing the pull of gravity, the Headstand redirects the flow of blood and lymph[4] throughout the entire body. Stagnant blood is drained from the legs, and the brain and upper endocrine glands are bathed in an increased supply of fresh, oxygen-rich blood. This pose benefits the entire nervous system, as well as the sense organs that are connected to the brain through the nerves. Scientific tests have shown that the Headstand improves memory and intellect.

---

[4] Lymph: a clear, yellowish fluid, containing white blood cells in a liquid resembling blood plasma, which is derived from the tissues of the body and conveyed to the blood stream by the lymphatic vessels.

This pose also aids digestion and elimination, alleviates urinary problems, tones internal organs, and reduces the risk of hernia and varicose veins. Because of these accumulated benefits, an overall sense of well-being is experienced by students who regularly practice this asana.

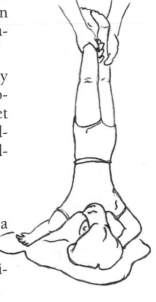

While the Preparation for the Headstand only inverts the body to a 45-degree angle, the Headstand completes this inversion process and brings the body perpendicular to the floor, with the feet directly above the head. As a result, the benefits of the full Headstand are much greater than those of the Preparation for the Headstand.

Technique:

1. Place your child on his back on top of a thick blanket or a large flat pillow.

2. Sit by your child's head in a kneeling or cross-legged position.

3. Reach out over his body and grasp his lower legs, just above the ankles.

4. Lift the legs off the floor.

5. Continue to lift, slowly bringing the her body into vertical alignment, with the top of her head lightly touching the floor. Try to keep the head in contact with the floor — this will provide a reference point to help him feel more secure.

6. Your child should now be completely upside down and facing you. Observe his face to see if he is comfortable and content to be in an inverted posture. If you notice the slightest degree of discomfort at any time, immediately bring him out of the pose.

7. Begin by holding the pose for 5 seconds and gradually work up to a maximum of one minute.

8. To bring him out of the pose, hold both legs with one of your hands and place your other hand at the back of his neck. Gently move his head toward you as you lower his legs.

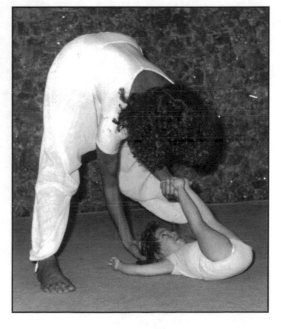

Variation:

Depending on the size of the child, you may find it easier to stand while assisting him in performing this pose (see following photo).

 Note:

(1) It is important to allow your child to rest on his back for at least one minute after performing the Headstand so that the blood pressure can equalize throughout his body. If you raise his head too soon, it may cause him to become faint.

(2) The Headstand is a more advanced pose and should not be introduced into your child's yoga routine until he is able to comfortably perform the Pre- paration for the Headstand for at least 30 seconds.

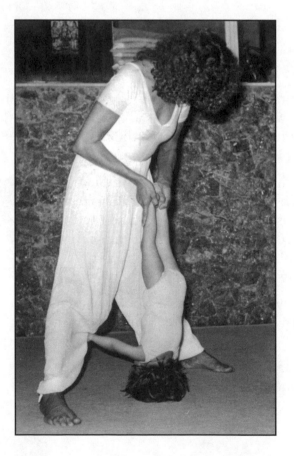

Conclusion to the Yoga Session

Deep Relaxation | Exercise 16

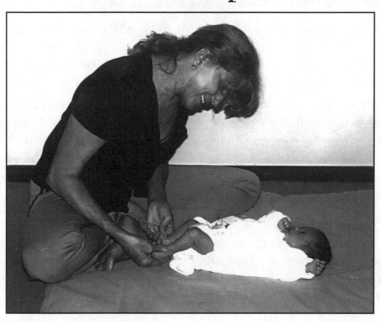

Benefits: Approximately 25 minutes have passed since the beginning of the yoga session, during which your child has had many areas of his stretched and toned. Now it is time for him to rest, in order to assimilate the benefits of all these movements and postures. In yoga, this is accomplished through Deep Relaxation. During Deep Relaxation, as muscles and nerves release stored-up tension, a sense of calm and focus is restored. The nervous system is strengthened and general health improves. For this reason, I recommend that you always include Deep Relaxation as an integral part of your child's yoga routine.

Technique:

During Deep Relaxation your child should be kept as comfortable and still as possible. Try not to make any sudden movements that might distract his attention from the interior process that is taking place. If you wish to speak, do so quietly and in a soothing tone of voice.

Having just completed the Headstand, your child should now be resting on his back. Prepare the room by dimming the lights and putting on a cassette or CD of quiet, relaxing music. If the room seems cool or drafty, cover him with a blanket. Sit at his feet and place them 6–12 inches apart. Begin the relaxation process by massaging both feet at the same time. Massage the soles, using your thumbs in a gentle kneading motion. Then massage the top of each foot with your fingers. Allow his legs to remain resting on the floor while you massage his feet.

Depending on the child, you may wish to continue working on his feet throughout the entire relaxation period, or you may decide to stop massaging after a few minutes. Some children respond positively if you massage them from feet to head, naming each part of the body as you work on it. This type of verbal communication can help to develop greater body awareness. Other children prefer to be massaged on the nape of the neck, the face, or the top of the head. If the child has difficulty relaxing on the floor, you can try cradling him in your arms. Sometimes the closeness of this type of physical contact helps to induce a state of relaxation.

Feel free to structure the relaxation period according to your own perception of your child's needs. By being positive, intuitive, affectionate, and loving, you will find the best way to help him relax. Don't worry if he falls asleep — he will continue to absorb the benefits of Deep Relaxation on a subconscious level. After approximately 10 minutes, bring your child out of Deep Relaxation by chanting or gently touching the soles of his feet. Finish the yoga session with some words of encouragement and (if you wish) several hugs and kisses.

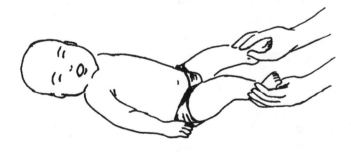

Notes and Comments on the Inductive Stage

- A complete yoga session, including Deep Relaxation, should last 30–35 minutes.

- Remember to allow time in between exercises for your child to relax in preparation for the next exercise.

- *If your child has seizures, suffers from a cardiac or spinal problem, or has had a recent illness or surgery, do not attempt to begin a program of yoga therapy without professional guidance.* You will need to contact a yoga teacher who is certified to practice the methods outlined in this book. The yoga teacher will be able to assess your child's needs and, in consultation with your physician, prepare a yoga program that your child can safely follow.

- Developing speech and language skills requires the assistance of a speech and/or language therapist. Yoga helps to improve respiration and will complement the work of the therapist.

- Remember that your child's enthusiasm and energy level can vary from time to time. Try to be sensitive to these changes and adjust the exercises accordingly.

- Be consistent. A little yoga every day will be much more effective in the long run than a lot of yoga once in a while.

Yoga Practice Chart for the Inductive Stage

Once you have become familiar with the Inductive Stage exercises, you may use the easy-reference chart at the end of this chapter to guide you through your child's yoga routine.

Inductive Stage Exercises

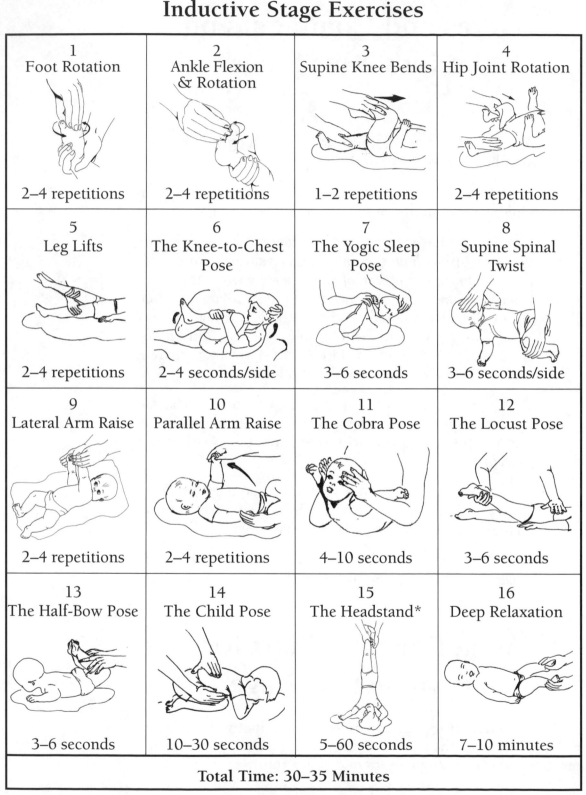

1 Foot Rotation	2 Ankle Flexion & Rotation	3 Supine Knee Bends	4 Hip Joint Rotation
2–4 repetitions	2–4 repetitions	1–2 repetitions	2–4 repetitions
5 Leg Lifts	6 The Knee-to-Chest Pose	7 The Yogic Sleep Pose	8 Supine Spinal Twist
2–4 repetitions	2–4 seconds/side	3–6 seconds	3–6 seconds/side
9 Lateral Arm Raise	10 Parallel Arm Raise	11 The Cobra Pose	12 The Locust Pose
2–4 repetitions	2–4 repetitions	4–10 seconds	3–6 seconds
13 The Half-Bow Pose	14 The Child Pose	15 The Headstand*	16 Deep Relaxation
3–6 seconds	10–30 seconds	5–60 seconds	7–10 minutes

Total Time: 30–35 Minutes

* The Headstand is a more advanced exercise and should not be attempted until the child can comfortably perform the Preparatory Stage version for a minimum of thirty seconds.

7

The Interactive Stage

Boosting the Level of Participation

(One to Two Years)

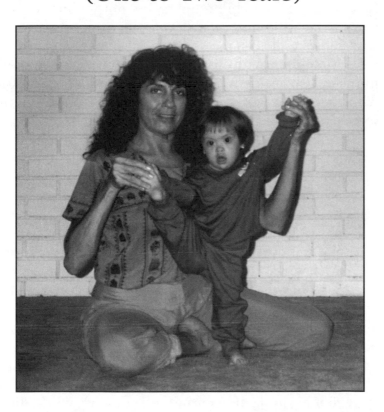

In order to begin practicing asanas in the Interactive Stage Program, your child should be able to sit alone and stand or walk with a minimum of assistance. With these newly acquired motor skills, she can begin to perform many of the more advanced asanas, including the seated, standing, and balancing poses. Initially, these asanas may be somewhat difficult for her to perform. The more she collaborates, however, the sooner she will succeed in mastering these poses. For this reason, you should encourage your child to increase her participation level during your practice sessions together.

As your child's participation level increases, so do the benefits of yoga therapy. These include: greater body awareness, a longer attention span, increased muscle tone, and improved circulation and lung capacity. Your child will demonstrate these gains during the yoga session as her movements become more graceful, fluid, and confident. At the same time, her need for your support and assistance will decrease. She will quickly learn to hold some of the poses without assistance, and others, with the touch of your hand. Your task at this time is to provide her with just enough help to go into and hold a given pose without strain or discomfort.

☑ **Note:** Infants (and children who are not mobile) characteristically lack the muscular development of older, more active children. Their bone density is also relatively low. In the case of children with disabilities, the joints are sometimes prone to displacement. Therefore, the parent or professional who chooses to work with an infant must be careful not to force or strain the child's body in any of the following exercises. Start with the minimum duration or number of repetitions specified for each exercise. As your child becomes accustomed to the exercises, you will be able to gradually increase these limits. Allow short rest periods between exercises as necessary.

Exercises having a greater degree of difficulty, such as the inverted, standing, or backward-bending poses are marked with an asterisk. These exercises, as well as the advanced variations of other exercises, should be incorporated into your child's practice only after she has demonstrated the ability to perform them without discomfort. On the other hand, if you feel she needs extra work on a specific area of her body, you should continue with the exercises for strengthening that area, even though they may be from an earlier stage. For example, if her arms and chest are weak, then she should continue performing the lateral and parallel arm raises until such time as her upper body strength increases. By staying attentive to your child's needs, you can help her avoid possible injury and achieve a progressive and well-rounded development.

Exercises From a Supine[1] Position

Exercises for the Feet and Ankles

Benefits: As in the Preparatory and Inductive Stages, one of the main objectives of the exercises in this section is to help prepare the child to stand and walk. These exercises promote strength and flexibility in the ankles and feet, help in the formation of the arches, and stimulate important energy points on the feet. The reason for starting with the feet is that they are the base for good posture when standing or walking. After performing these exercises, you may spend a few minutes massaging your child's feet. The relaxing effects of this massage will help to prepare her for the exercises that follow.

---

[1] Supine: lying on the back.

Exercise 1 | Foot Rotation

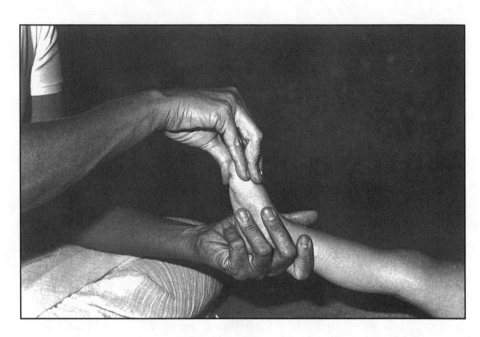

Technique:

1. Gently place your child on her back.

2. Take a comfortable seated position at her feet and place one of her heels in the palm of your upturned hand.

3. Wrap your fingers around the heel so that your thumb is pressing against one side of the ankle and your four fingers are pressing on the other side. This should secure the heel and immobilize the ankle joint.

4. With the other hand, hold the toes of the same foot and make circular movements with the upper part of the foot, first clockwise, then counterclockwise.

5. Do 2–4 repetitions in each direction and repeat with the other foot.

☑ **Note:** If your child's foot has a tendency to bend either inward or outward, any movement that puts pressure in the same direction will increase this tendency. If you emphasize movements in the opposite direction, the problem will be alleviated.

Ankle Flexion and Rotation | Exercise 2

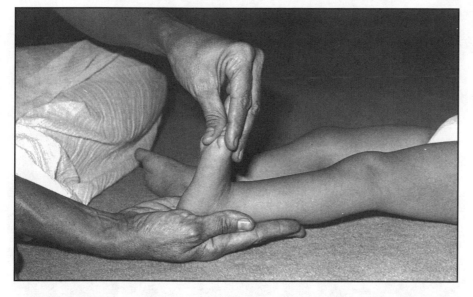

Technique:

1. Sit at your child's feet.

2. Hold one of her legs directly above the ankle.

3. Grasp the toes of the same foot with the tips of the fingers of your other hand.

4. Gently bend the toes and foot, first upward (away from you), then downward (toward you).

5. Do 2–4 repetitions and repeat with the other foot.

6. Make circular movements with the toes, first clockwise, then counterclockwise.

7. Do 2–4 repetitions in each direction and repeat the entire exercise with the other foot.

☑ **Note:**

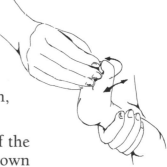

(1) If your child's foot has a tendency to bend either inward or outward, any movement that puts pressure in the same direction will increase this tendency. If you emphasize movements in the opposite direction, the problem will be alleviated.

(2) Follow Exercises 1 and 2 by massaging the soles of the feet. Use your thumbs in a kneading motion, working down from the toes to the heels of each foot. Be sure to include the inside arch of the foot.

Exercises for the Legs and Hips

Exercise

3

Supine Knee Bends

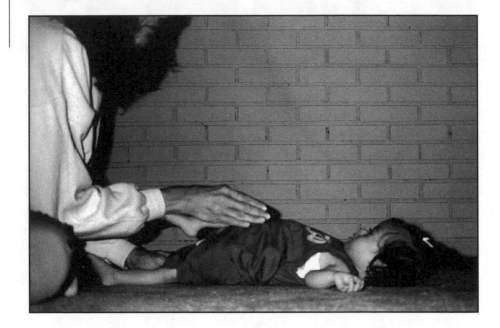

Benefits: This exercise increases flexibility in the knees and hips, relieves tension in the lower back, and strengthens the tendons, nerves, and musculature of the legs. It also has a stimulating effect on the organs of the abdomen and helps to relieve gas, colic, and constipation.

Technique:

1. Sit at your child's feet.

2. Place your left hand on top of her right thigh.

3. With your right hand, grasp the top of her left leg directly below the knee.

4. Slowly raise the left leg off the floor, allowing the knee to flex at the same time. Use your left hand to help stabilize her body, making sure that the right leg remains flat on the floor.

5. Push gently against the raised leg to increase the flexion in the knee. As you do so, the knee will pivot up over the hips, and the thigh will approach, or possibly even touch, the chest. Stop

at the point where you feel resistance. Do not attempt to force the leg beyond this point.

6. Slowly return the left leg to its original position.

7. Do 1–2 repetitions and repeat with the other leg. Then perform the same exercise with both legs at the same time.

☑ **Note:**

(1) Make sure your child's body retains its alignment during all phases of this exercise by keeping both hips on the floor and the raised leg(s) from tilting either to the right or to the left.

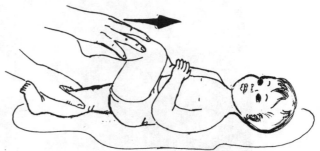

(2) The goal of this exercise is to be able to touch your child's thigh to her chest. If you work slowly and patiently, the range of motion in the hip joint will gradually increase.

☒ **Caution:** If your child has had a colostomy, watch closely to make sure that she is not experiencing any discomfort. If necessary, reduce the degree of movement until you find an appropriate comfort level for performing this exercise.

Exercise 4 | *Pedaling*

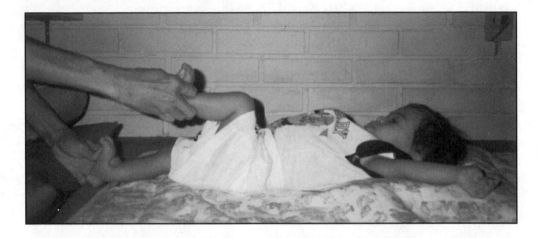

Benefits: This repetitive exercise tones the thighs and overall musculature of the legs. Its rapid movements work the knee and hip joints and help to increase circulation and motor coordination in the legs. The exercise also helps to relieve gas and constipation.

Technique:

1. Sit at your child's feet.

2. Grasp her left foot with your right hand, and her right foot with your left hand. Now raise her extended legs approximately six inches off the floor.

3. Push her right foot away from you, allowing the knee to flex and raising the thigh into a vertical position.

4. Perform the same movement with her left leg while pulling the right leg back to its original position.

5. Continue to pump her legs as if she were pedaling a bicycle. The total time for this exercise should be approximately 30 seconds.

 Note: For maximum stability, make sure both hips remain on the floor during this exercise.

The Leg Lift Pose | Exercise 5

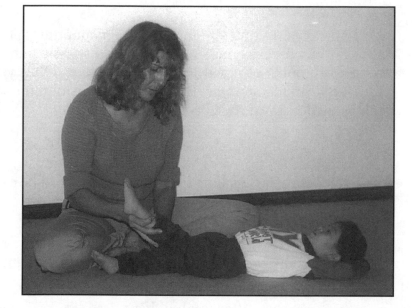

Benefits: This exercise strengthens the muscles of the abdomen and thighs. It also elongates the hamstrings and posterior muscles of the legs. The advanced variation provides a powerful forward-bending stretch that works the muscles of the arms, chest, and neck.

Technique:

1. Sit at your child's feet.

2. Place your right hand on the outside of her left knee. The fingers of your right hand should now be resting on top of her left knee, with your thumb extending beneath the calf of her leg.

3. Using your thumb and fingers to keep her knee from bending, raise her leg off the floor to a 90-degree angle. Continue the movement over her hips and toward her chest. Keep the other leg on the floor with your left hand.

4. Hold this position momentarily, then return the right leg to the floor.

5. Do 2–4 repetitions and repeat with the other leg. Then perform the same exercise with both legs at the same time.

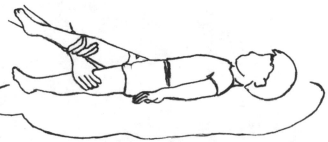

(1) Make sure both of your child's hips remain on the floor during all phases of this exercise.

(2) Work toward gradually increasing the amount of time spent in the raised-leg position. As you do so, you can decrease the number of repetitions of the exercise. Once your child is able to maintain her leg in a raised position for several seconds, this exercise becomes an asana.

(3) As your child gains more upper body strength, she will be able to raise her legs with less assistance on your part. The greater her participation, the more her muscles will be exercised.

Advanced Variation:

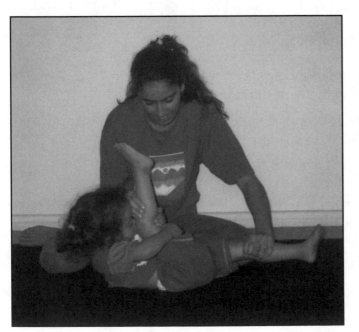

1. Sit alongside your child and perform Steps 2 and 3.

2. Ask your child to reach up with both hands and grasp the calf or thigh of her raised leg. Wait a few seconds, then give her just enough help to perform these movements.

3. Ask her to try to raise her head up toward her raised leg. Wait a few seconds, then give her just enough help to perform this movement.

4. Hold this pose for 1–2 seconds.

5. To help her come out of the pose, slowly lower her body in reverse order, beginning with the head, then the arms, and finally the legs.

6. Repeat the same sequence with the other leg, and then with both legs at the same time.

Exercises for Strengthening the Muscles of the Abdomen

The Forward Boat Pose

Exercise

6

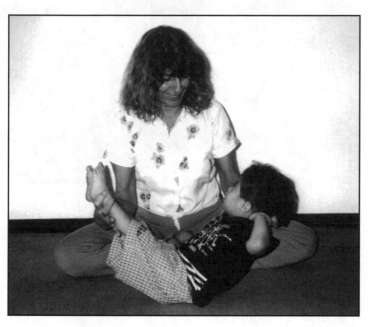

Benefits: The Forward Boat Pose is excellent for developing balance and strengthening the muscles of the abdomen, chest, shoulders, neck, and thighs. It also helps to elongate the spine and tone the abdominal organs.

Technique:

1. Sit alongside your child, facing her midsection.

2. Place one hand beneath both ankles and the other hand beneath the back of her neck.

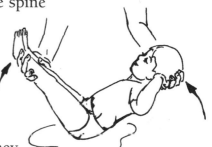

3. Simultaneously raise the upper body and legs until they form a "V," with each side of the "V" at a 45-degree angle from the floor.

4. Hold this position for 5–10 seconds.

5. To help her come out of the pose, slowly lower her upper body and legs to the floor.

☑ **Note:** As your child's abdominal muscles and thighs become stronger you will be able to gradually reduce your support beneath her neck and ankles.

Exercise 7 | *Sit Ups**

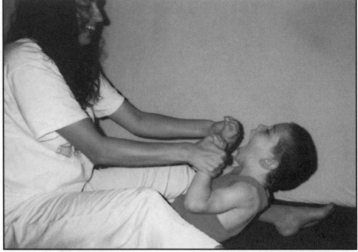

Benefits: This repetitive exercise tones the muscles of the thighs, abdomen, chest, arms, and neck. It is especially beneficial for strengthening the muscles of the abdomen.

Technique:

1. Place a large pillow or thick cushion beneath your child's upper back, neck, and head.

2. Sit at her feet.

3. Place one hand on top of her legs and the other hand above her chest. Depending on the child, you may need to secure her legs by overlapping them with your own (see photo and drawing).

4. Ask her to reach up with both hands and grasp your extended hand. Once she has a firm grip, pull her arms toward you until her upper body is vertical. Use your other hand to keep her legs from lifting off the floor.

5. Lower her down to the cushion to complete one repetition. Repeat 5–10 times.

☑ **Note:** Once your child becomes accustomed to performing this exercise, encourage her to sit up with less assistance. Eventually she will be able to sit up completely on her own.

---

*Asterisk-marked exercises should be incorporated into your child's practice only after she has demonstrated the ability to perform them without discomfort.

Exercises for the Torso

The Bridge Pose | *Exercise* 8

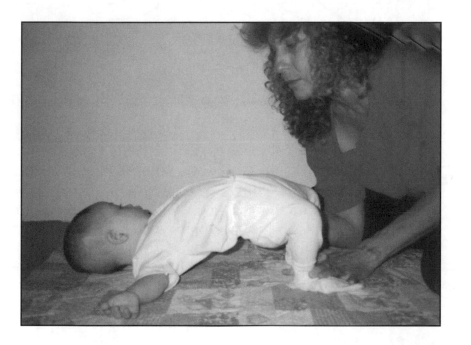

Benefits: This pose stretches the hip joints and the lumbar area of the back. It also strengthens the muscles of the lower back, buttocks, and thighs.

Technique:

1. Sit at your child's feet.

2. Bend her legs at the knees and place both feet flat on the floor. Position the feet approximately three inches apart.

3. Place one of your hands over her feet and the other, palm up, beneath the small of her back.

4. Hold both feet firmly on the floor. Raise her back off the floor until her body forms an arch, beginning at the feet and ending at the shoulders.

5. Hold this pose for 3–5 seconds.

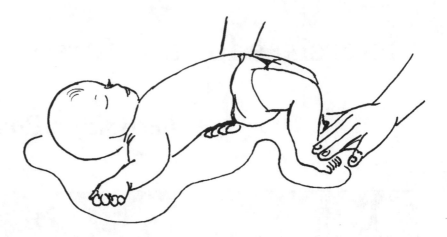

6. To help her come out of the pose, slowly lower her back and legs to the floor.

☑ **Note:** A time will come when your child will be able to raise her hips off the floor without your help. You can encourage her to work toward this goal in the following manner: Begin the exercise by placing her feet approximately six inches apart for greater stability. Ask her to lift her hips off the floor without offering any assistance. After a few seconds, give her just enough support beneath the lower back to complete the pose.

The Knee-to-Chest Pose | *Exercise* 9

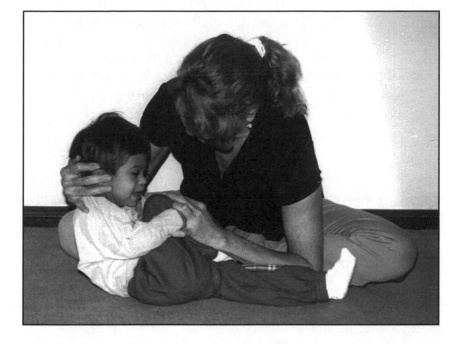

Benefits: This asana is excellent for relieving gas, colic, and other intestinal problems. It strengthens the muscles of the abdomen, stretches muscles of the back and neck, and helps to increase flexibility in the hips and knees. It is especially beneficial for relieving stress in the lower back.

Technique:

1. Sit to the left side of your child.

2. Place your right hand on top of her left thigh. Place your left hand on top of her right leg directly below the knee.

3. Grasp the right leg and raise it off the floor, allowing the knee to flex at the same time. Push gently against the leg to increase the flexion in the knee.

4. Replace your left hand with your right hand and lower your right forearm until it rests on top of her leg. During the remainder of this exercise, you can use your right forearm to keep the left leg from lifting off the floor.

5. With your right hand, continue to push gently against the child's right leg. As you do so, the knee will pivot up over the

hips, and the thigh will approach, or possibly even touch, the chest.

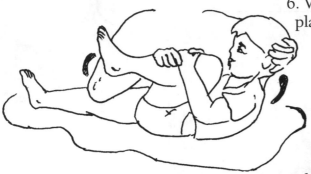

6. Without offering any assistance, ask her to place her hands on top of her bent knee. Wait a few seconds, then give her just enough help (with your left hand) to perform these movements. Secure both of her hands with your right hand.

7. Ask her to raise her head toward her knee. After a few seconds, reach under the back of her head (with your left hand) and give her just enough help to perform this movement. Raise her head as far as you can without discomfort, endeavoring to touch her chin or forehead to the knee. As you do so, she will naturally exhale.

8. Hold this position until you feel her begin to inhale (about 2–4 seconds).

9. To help her come out of the pose, lower her head first, then the arms and leg to the floor.

10. Repeat this exercise with the other leg. Then perform it with both legs at the same time.

 Note: Make sure your child's body retains its alignment during all phases of this exercise by keeping both hips on the floor and the raised leg(s) from tilting either to the right or to the left .

Caution: Remember to reduce the degree of movement and duration of the pose if your child has had a colostomy.

The Yogic Sleep Pose | Exercise 10

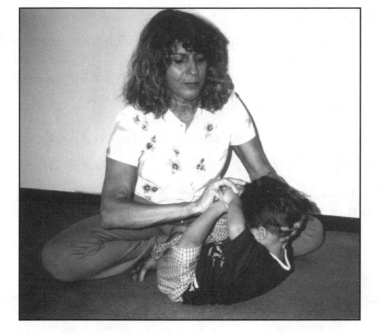

Benefits: This pose creates a forward-bending stretch along the entire spine. It also tones the organs of the abdomen and helps to increase mobility in the hips and knees.

Technique:

1. Sit to the right side of your child.

2. Grasp both ankles and raise her legs off the floor until they are vertical.

3. With one hand on each ankle, separate the ankles and bring the soles of the feet together above the child's body. In order to accomplish this, you will need to lower both feet toward the chest, allowing the knees to bend outward in opposite directions.

4. Clasp both feet together with your right hand and ask her to reach up and grab her feet. Wait a few seconds and then, with your free hand, give her just enough help to perform these movements.

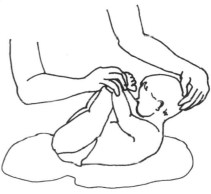

5. Holding both hands and both feet together with your right hand, ask her to raise her head up toward her feet. After a few seconds reach

under the back of her neck with your left hand and give her just enough help to perform this movement. Try to touch her forehead to her feet. The hands, feet, and forehead should ideally meet at a single point.

6. Hold this position until you feel the child begin to inhale (about 3–6 seconds).

7. To help her come out of the pose, lower the head first, then the arms and legs to the floor.

 Note: Make sure both of your child's hips remain on the floor during all phases of this exercise.

 Caution: Remember to reduce the degree of movement and duration of the pose if your child has had a colostomy.

Exercises from a Prone² Position

Backward-Bending Poses

Backward-bending poses form one of the four basic groups of asanas for the spine. The other three groups are forward-bending, twisting, and side-bending poses. The backward-bending poses reverse the stretch of the forward-bending poses; a left twist reverses the stretch of a right twist, and so on. Taken together, all four groups constitute a total program for keeping the spinal column flexible, healthy, and resilient. These complementary poses fortify the central nervous system, strengthen and elongate all the muscles of the torso, and benefit all the internal organs.

---

² Prone: lying with the front or face downward.

The Swan Pose* | Exercise 11

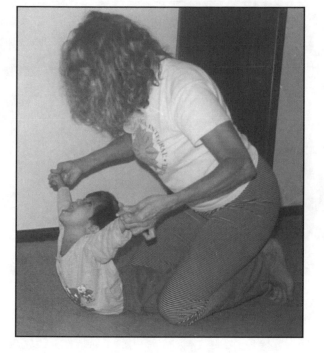

Benefits: This asana releases tension from the lower back, strengthens upper back and neck muscles, expands the rib cage, and relieves constipation and gas.

Technique:

1. Gently turn your child onto her stomach.

2. Kneel down with your knees positioned on either side of her legs.

3. Reach out and grasp both of her hands, stretching the arms in opposite directions.

4. Lift her outstretched arms upward, so that her head, neck, chest, and abdomen rise off the floor. Make sure the pelvis remains on the floor.

5. Hold for 3–6 seconds.

6. To help her come out of the pose, slowly lower her outstretched arms to the floor.

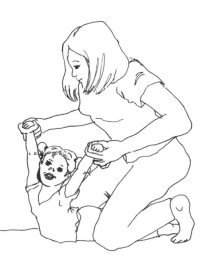

*The Cobra Pose**

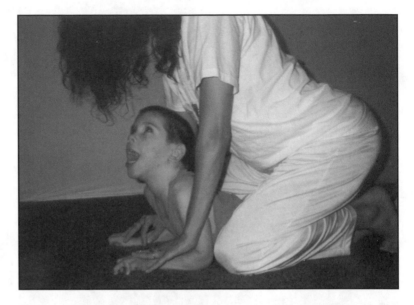

⊠ **Caution:** Do not allow your child to straighten her arms in the Cobra Pose if she has lordosis or any other type of lower back problem.

Benefits: Similar to the Swan Pose, the Cobra Pose requires a greater degree of muscular development in the neck, shoulders, arms, and upper back. This asana elongates the body's anterior muscles and helps to release tension from the solar plexus and lower back. It expands the rib cage, tones the heart, lungs, and cranial nerves, and strengthens the upper back and neck muscles. It also helps to correct spinal misalignment and to relieve constipation and gas. The Swan Pose and Push-Up Pose, as well as the Parallel and Lateral Arm Raises, will help prepare the child to perform the Cobra Pose.

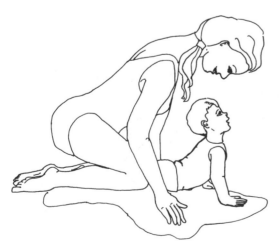

Technique:

1. Kneel down with your knees positioned on either side of your child's legs.

2. Place her hands on the floor directly beneath her shoulders. Make sure her fingers are pointing forward, with the palms down and the bent elbows alongside the body. Secure

her hands in this position by holding them with both of your hands.

3. Straighten your arms, come up on your knees, and center your head directly over the child's head.

4. Call out her name or say something that will attract her attention. This will prompt her to push down on the floor with her hands, raise her head, and look up.

5. Stay centered above her head, so that she will continue to move it upward and backward. With this method, you will be able to encourage the child to raise her entire upper body off the floor and eventually straighten both arms.

6. Allow her to hold the pose as long as she is comfortable. She will come out of the pose when ready (3–30 seconds).

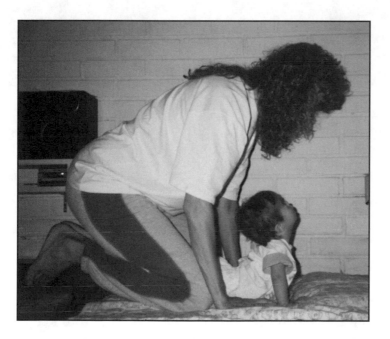

The Locust Pose

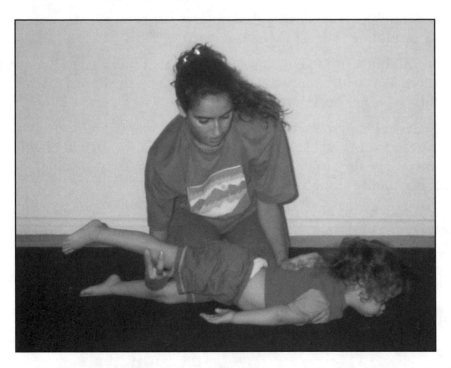

Benefits: This asana strengthens the muscles of the lower back and buttocks, stretches the abdominal muscles, and tones the organs and glands of the abdomen.

Technique:

1. Sit to the left side of your child.

2. Bring her legs together and position her arms alongside her body.

3. Place the palm of your left hand on her lower back.

4. With your right hand underneath her left knee, slowly raise her extended leg off the floor. Use your left hand to keep her left hip on the floor.

5. Stop at the point of resistance and hold the pose for 3–6 seconds.

6. To help her come out of the pose, slowly lower her leg to the floor.

7. Repeat the Locust Pose with the other leg. Then perform the same exercise with both legs at the same time.

Advanced Variation:

1. Sit at your child's feet.

2. Grasp both of her ankles with your left hand and place your right hand (palm up) beneath her knees.

3. Raise her legs, using your right hand to keep the knees from bending. Start by raising only the legs off the floor. As the child's flexibility develops, you can increase the stretch until the hips also lift off the floor.

4. Hold the pose for 3–6 seconds.

5. To help her come out of the pose, slowly lower her legs to the floor.

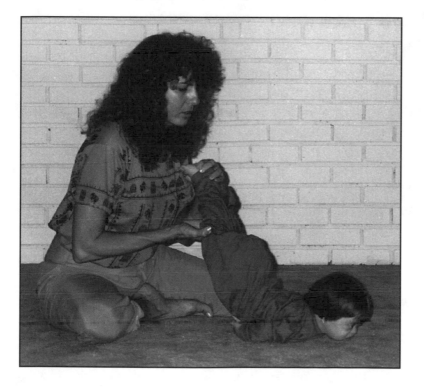

The Bow Pose* | Exercise 14

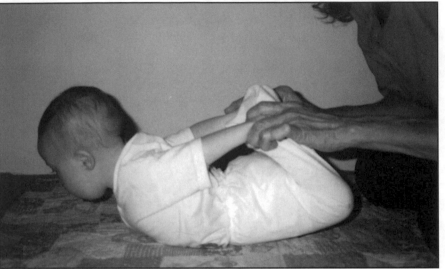

Caution: Do not perform this exercise if your child has lordosis or any other type of lower back problem.

Benefits: This asana elongates the thigh muscles and provides many of the same benefits as both the Cobra and Locust Poses. In addition, the Bow Pose reduces abdominal fat, stimulates the pancreas, and increases peristalsis in the large intestine.

Technique:

1. Sit at your child's feet.

2. Grasp the child's ankles and raise them off the floor, allowing the knees to bend.

3. Hold her feet together with one of your hands.

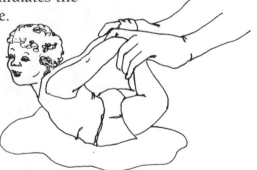

4. Reach out with your free hand and bring her hands, one at a time, back to her feet.

5. Grasp her right hand and right foot with your right hand, and her left hand and left foot with your left hand. You should now be holding both hands and both feet close together above her back.

6. Raise her hands and feet so that her chest and thighs come off the floor.

7. Hold the pose for 3–6 seconds.

8. To help her come out of the pose, slowly lower her chest and thighs, and then return her arms and legs to the floor.

The Push-Up Pose* | Exercise 15

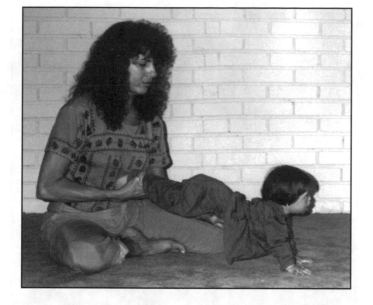

Benefits: This pose strengthens the muscles of the arms, shoulders, neck, and back.

Technique:

1. Sit at your child's feet.

2. Place her hands on the floor directly beneath her shoulders.

3. Grasp her lower legs with one of your hands and place the other (palm up) beneath her chest.

4. Keeping her legs straight, raise them about six inches off the floor.

5. Ask your child to push her upper body off the floor. Give her just enough support so she can perform this movement.

6. Continue assisting her until both arms are fully extended. As you do so, lift her legs higher until they are 1–1½ feet off the floor. Try to keep the trunk and legs in a straight line.

7. Hold for 3–6 seconds.

8. To help her come out of the pose, slowly lower her trunk and legs to the floor.

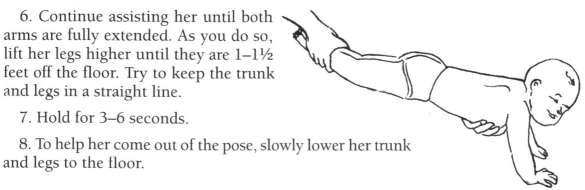

Exercise 16 | The Child Pose

Benefits: This pose reverses the stretch of the previous backward-bending poses. It creates a gentle forward-bending stretch that helps to elongate the spine and reduce disk compression, especially in the lower back. Like the Knee-to-Chest Pose, it helps to relieve colic, gas, and other intestinal problems.

Technique:

1. Sit at your child's feet.

2. Place one of your hands over both of her calves and the other hand (palm up) beneath her chest.

3. Hold the calves down and raise the chest off the floor.

4. Use Your upturned hand to move her chest back toward her feet. As you do this, her knees will bend, and her hips will pivot up over the knees and down toward the floor. Continue the movement until her buttocks are resting on her heels.

5. Lower her chest onto her thighs. Remove your hands and adjust both feet so that the soles are facing upward.

6. Help her maintain this position by placing one of your hands on her lower back and exerting a gentle downward pressure.

7. Hold this posture until you feel her trying to extend her legs (10–30 seconds).

8. To help her come out of the pose, place one hand over her calves and the other beneath her chest. Then return her upper body to a prone position.

☑ **Note:** To exercise the muscles of her neck, ask your child to raise her head off the floor while in the Child Pose.

Advanced Variation:

Benefits: This important variation will develop your child's balance and train her to sit, crawl, and stand.

Technique:

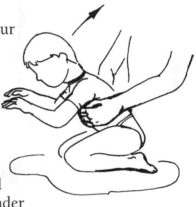

1. From the Child Pose, place one of your hands (palm up) beneath your child's chest and the other (palm down) against the center of her upper back.

2. Raise her upper body into a vertical position, maintaining her balance with your hands. The child should now be sitting up with her lower legs folded under her and her buttocks resting on her heels. This position is called the Pelvic Pose.

3. Move your hands down from her chest and upper back to just above either hip. Use your hands to stabilize her hips while she works to keep her upper body erect.

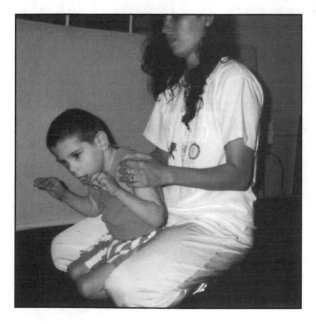

4. Hold this position for 10–20 seconds, before allowing her to return to the Child Pose.

Exercises from a Seated Position

Exercise 17 | *The Spinal Twist*

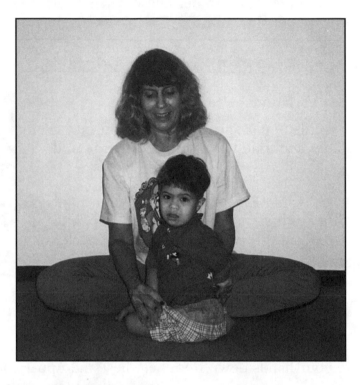

Benefits: The twisting movements of this asana stretch the connecting ligaments of the vertebrae, reduce disk compression, and stimulate nerves and ganglia in the area surrounding the spine. By compressing first one side of the body and then the other, this exercise massages and tones internal organs and glands, benefiting the liver, spleen, pancreas, kidneys, and adrenals. It also helps to relieve muscular tension in the back, waist, and hips. Because this pose is performed in an upright seated posture, as opposed to a supine position (see Supine Spinal Twist in Chapters 5 and 6), it has a much greater toning effect on the muscles of the arms, shoulders, and lower back, as well as on the organs of the abdomen.

Technique:

1. Sit your child up in a comfortable cross-legged position with her back toward you. Adjust her posture to make sure her back is straight.

2. Hold both arms and twist her trunk to the right, using the arms as levers to accomplish this movement.

3. To complete the twist, ask her to also turn her head to the right. Keep the body upright and stable during this pose.

4. Hold for 3–6 seconds.

5. To help her come out of the pose, slowly reverse the twist until she is facing forward. Then repeat the Spinal Twist in the opposite direction.

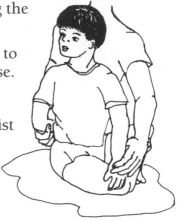

Forward-Bending Poses

The Head-to-Knee Pose | *Exercise* *18*

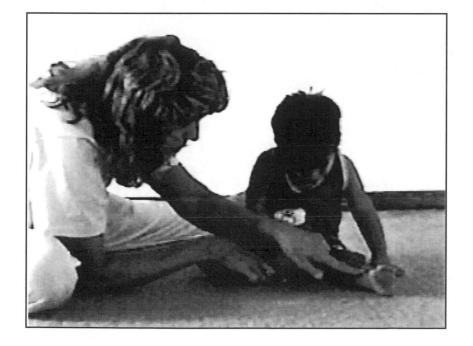

Benefits: Regular practice of the Head-to-Knee Pose helps to release tension in the lower back and to prevent constipation. This asana prepares your child for the Forward Bend.

Technique:

1. Sit behind your child, who should still be seated in a cross-legged position.

2. Extend one of her legs directly in front of her body.

3. Adjust the other leg so that her knee is on the floor and the sole of her foot is touching the inner thigh of her extended leg. Move her heel up to her perineum.

4. Ask her to reach out over her extended leg and grasp the ankle or foot with both hands.

5. Then ask her to bend forward and try to touch her forehead to her lower leg or ankle. Provide whatever assistance she may need to lower her body toward her leg.

6. Hold the pose for 5–15 seconds.

7. To help her come out of the pose, ask her to sit up. Then repeat the Head-to-Knee Pose with her other leg.

☑ Note: Keep her extended leg as straight as possible during this exercise.

The Forward Bend | *Exercise* 19

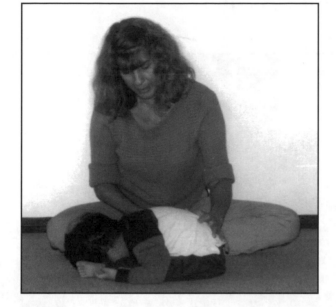

Benefits: The Forward Bend helps to elongate the spinal column by stretching the muscles and ligaments attached to the vertebrae. It gives an excellent stretch to all the posterior muscles. This asana benefits the entire body, especially the central nervous system. It tones the organs of the abdomen and helps to relieve tension in the lower back.

Technique:

1. Sit facing your child.

2. Extend both of her legs in front of her, bringing the feet together.

3. Ask her to reach out over her extended legs and grasp her ankles or feet.

4. Then ask her to bend forward and try to touch her forehead to her lower legs or ankles. If she is really limber, she may even be able to touch her chest to her thighs. Provide whatever assistance she may need to lower her body toward her legs.

5. Hold the pose for 5–15 seconds.

6. To help her come out of the pose, ask her to sit up.

☑ **Note:** Keep the child's extended legs as straight as possible during this exercise.

Exercise 20

The Forward Bend
(With Legs Apart)

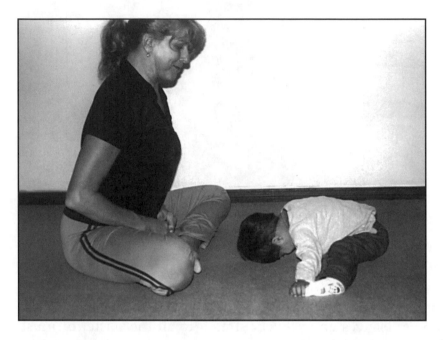

Benefits: This pose is excellent for limbering the hips and elongating the hamstrings and tendons of the inner thighs.

Technique:

1. Sit facing your child.

2. Extend both of her legs in front of her.

3. Gently move the legs apart until they form a wide "V."

4. Hold her ankles to keep the legs from moving together. Ask her to bend forward and try to lower her forehead to the floor. If she places her hands on the floor in front of her, she will be able to support herself as she lowers her body toward the floor. Provide whatever assistance she may need to perform this movement.

5. If she is able to reach the floor with her forehead or chest, you can spread her arms apart and place her hands on her ankles.

6. Hold the pose for 5–15 seconds.

7. To help her come out of the pose, raise her torso up to a seated position.

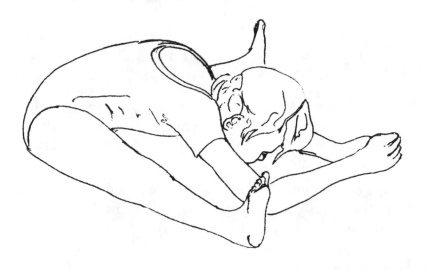

☑ **Note:** The Forward Bend (With Legs Apart) provides an intense stretch to the inner thighs. To avoid cramps and strains, start slowly and be sure not to force your child's legs.

Exercises from a Standing Position

Exercise

21

Standing Poses*

Benefits: Standing poses develop muscular strength and teach your child balance, body awareness, and concentration. Practiced regularly, these asanas are excellent training tools for learning to stand alone and walk.

Begin working with the Tree Pose. When your child is able to perform this pose, you can experiment with the Standing Knee-to-Chest Pose.

21-1 | ## The Tree Pose

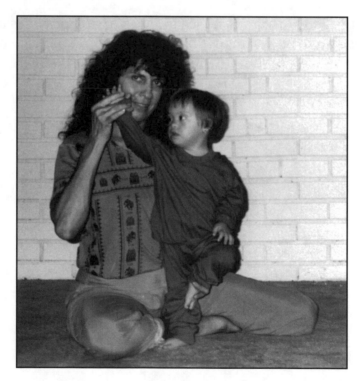

Technique:

1. Help your child onto her feet.

2. Sit or kneel behind her and wrap your left arm around her chest for support.

3. With your right hand, grasp the calf of her right leg and lift the leg just enough so that you can rotate the hip and bent knee out to the side. Place the sole of her right foot on the inside of her left leg, directly above the ankle.

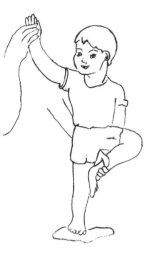

4. Hold the pose for 3–10 seconds.

5. To help her come out of the pose, lower her right foot to the floor. Then repeat the Tree Pose with the other leg.

☑ Note: There are several variations of the Tree Pose, depending on where your child places her foot on the supporting leg. The higher she places her foot, the more skill she will need to perform the pose.

The Standing Knee-to-Chest Pose | 21-2

Technique:

1. Help your child onto her feet.

2. Sit or kneel behind her and wrap your left arm around her chest for support.

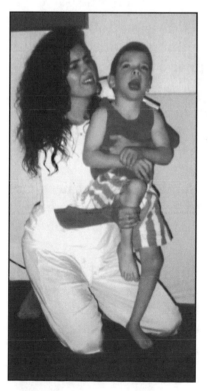

3. With your right hand, grasp her right leg just below the knee and raise it up toward her chest. The bent leg should be directly in front of the child's body.

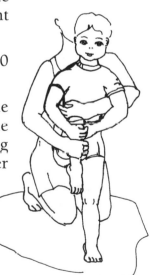

4. Hold the pose for 3–10 seconds.

5. To help her come out of the pose, lower her right foot to the floor. Then repeat the Standing Knee-to-Chest Pose with the other leg.

Exercise 22

Standing Forward Bends*

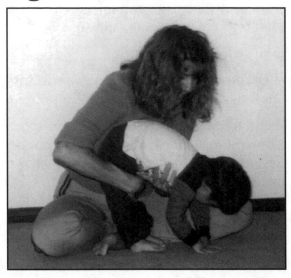

Benefits: This repetitive exercise is excellent for developing strength in the back and legs.

Technique:

1. Remain seated behind your child.

2. Wrap one arm around the front of the child's knees.

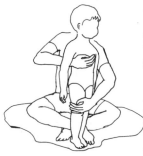

3. Ask her to bend forward as far as possible and place both hands on the floor. Use your free hand to support her chest as she bends forward and lowers her upper body toward the floor.

4. Ask her to return to an upright position. With your hand on her chest, give her just enough support to perform this movement.

5. Repeat 1–5 times.

☑ **Note:**

1) In the beginning, until your child develops greater muscular strength, she will be able to perform only one or two repetitions of this exercise. Gradually increase the number to a maximum of 5 repetitions.

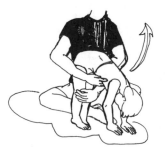

2) Some children may feel apprehensive about bending forward the first few times they perform this exercise. One way to deal with this problem is by placing an object on the floor several feet in front of your child. Ask her to pick up the object and give it to you. Making a game out of the exercise will help her to forget her fear.

Inverted Poses

☑ **Note:** Generally, it is sufficient for your child to perform one inverted pose per yoga session. The Headstand is provided as an option to the Shoulder Stand (and Fish Pose). You may alternate these two inverted poses from session to session. You may also work with one pose for a period of several days or weeks depending on the child's specific needs and receptivity.

*The Shoulder Stand** | *Exercise* 23

☒ **Caution:** If your child is on medication, check with your pharmacist or pediatrician to make sure that it is safe to place the child in an inverted position. If your child has a cardiac problem or seizures, then you should contact a yoga teacher who is certified to practice the methods outlined in this book. The yoga teacher will be able to assess your child's needs and, in consultation with your physician, prepare a yoga program that your child can safely follow. In addition, because the Shoulder Stand flexes the cervical vertebrae, it should not be performed by children with atlanto-axial instability.[3] This orthopedic problem affects 10–20 percent of children with Down

---

[3] Atlanto-axial instability is a condition of increased mobility in the joint between the atlas and the axis, the two cervical vertebrae at the base of the skull.

Syndrome. Check with your pediatrician to make sure that your child does not have this condition.

Benefits: Known as the "Queen of Asanas," the Shoulder Stand is one of two inverted poses that form an integral part of almost every yoga routine. Like the Headstand, the Shoulder Stand reverses the pull of gravity and redirects the flow of blood and lymph[4] throughout the entire body. Stagnant blood is drained from the legs, and the brain and upper endocrine glands are bathed in an increased supply of fresh, oxygen-rich blood. This pose aids digestion and elimination and alleviates asthma, throat, and urinary problems. It also tones internal organs and reduces the risk of hernias and varicose veins.

While the Headstand provides greater benefit for the pituitary and pineal glands, the Shoulder Stand concentrates its benefits in the thyroid and parathyroid glands, which regulate the body's metabolism. This asana stretches the muscles and ligaments attached to the cervical vertebrae, and strengthens the muscles of the shoulders, arms, and back.

Technique:

1. Place your child on her back.

2. Sit at her feet in a comfortable cross-legged position.

3. Grasp her ankles and pull her body toward you, lifting upward as you pull. Continue to pull and lift until her legs are level with your chest and her back is resting against your abdomen. At this point, she should be in an inverted position with her shoulders, arms, neck, and head touching the floor.

4. Hold the pose for 30–60 seconds.

5. To come out of the pose, hold both her ankles with one hand and place your free hand beneath the small of her back. Raise the back just enough to slide her body away from you, lowering her legs at the same time.

Variations: Once your child is comfortable in the Shoulder Stand, you can introduce several

---

[4] Lymph: a clear, yellowish fluid, containing white blood cells in a liquid resembling blood plasma, which is derived from the tissues of the body and conveyed to the blood stream by the lymphatic vessels.

variations. These variations stretch and strengthen the legs, back, and neck, increase mobility in the hip joints, and improve balance and body awareness. Begin with Variation 1, and add Variations 2 and 3 as your child becomes accustomed to performing each successive variation.

Variation 1: Leg Splits

1. From the Shoulder Stand, grasp the outside of each calf and move your child's legs apart until they form a wide "V."

2. Bring the legs back together.

3. Repeat 1–3 times.

Variation 2: Leg Lifts

1. Grasp the outside of each calf and lower your child's right leg to the floor behind her head. Make sure that her legs remain straight during this movement.

2. Return her right leg to a vertical position.

3. Perform the same movements with her left leg.

4. Repeat 1–3 times.

Variation 3: The Plow Pose

1. Grasp the outside of each calf and slowly lower your child's extended legs to the floor behind her head.

2. Return the legs to a vertical position.

3. Repeat 1–3 times.

☑ Note:

1) In Variations 2 and 3, be careful not to strain your child's neck or upper back as you lower her legs down to the floor.

2) Once your child has sufficient control over her hip, leg, and back movements, encourage her to perform the Shoulder Stand variations without your assistance.

Exercise 24 | The Fish Pose

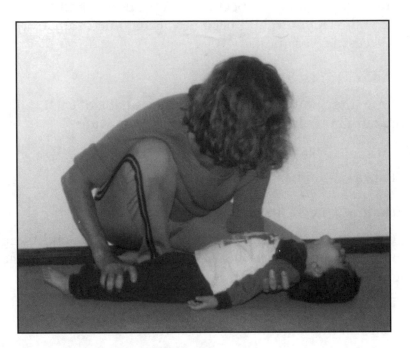

❌ **Caution:** Because the Fish Pose flexes the cervical vertebrae, it should not be performed by children with atlanto-axial instability. Check with your pediatrician to make sure that your child does not have this condition.

Benefits: This asana is the traditional counter-pose to the Shoulder Stand, opening areas of the neck and chest that were compressed in the inverted posture. Practicing the Fish Pose directly after the Shoulder Stand helps to relieve stiffness in the neck and shoulders. It complements the Shoulder Stand's benefits to the nervous system and upper endocrine glands, especially the thyroid.

Technique:

1. Your child should now be resting on her back, after having just completed the Shoulder Stand.

2. Sit by her side, facing her mid-section.

3. Raise her back off the floor just enough to slide one of your hands, palm up, beneath her upper back at the base of her neck.

4. Use your upturned hand to lift her back, neck, and head off the floor.

5. Place your free hand on her forehead. Very gently lower her forehead down until the top of her head is resting lightly on the floor. Her torso should now form an arch with only her buttocks and top of her head touching the floor.

6. Hold the pose for 5–10 seconds while continuing to support her upper back.

7. To help her come out of the pose, place your free hand beneath the back of her head. Raise her head slightly, and slowly lower her back and head to the floor.

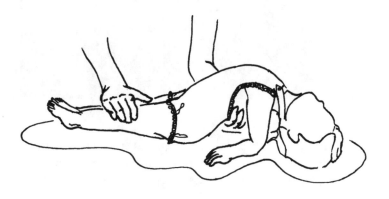

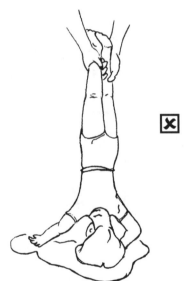

Exercise 25 | *The Headstand**

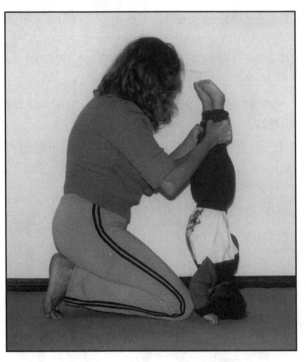

Caution: If your child is on medication, check with your pharmacist or pediatrician to make sure that it is safe to place the child in an inverted position. If your child has a cardiac problem or seizures, then you should contact a yoga teacher who is certified to practice the methods outlined in this book. The yoga teacher will be able to assess your child's needs and, in consultation with your physician, prepare a yoga program that your child can safely follow.

Benefits: By reversing the pull of gravity, the Headstand redirects the flow of blood and lymph throughout the entire body. Stagnant blood is drained from the legs, and the brain and upper endocrine glands are bathed in an increased supply of fresh, oxygen-rich blood. This pose benefits the entire nervous system, as well as the sense organs that are connected to the brain through the nerves. Scientific tests have shown that the Headstand improves memory and intellect.

This pose also aids digestion and elimination, alleviates urinary problems, tones internal organs, and reduces the risk of hernia and varicose veins. Because of these accumulated benefits, an overall sense of well-being is experienced by students who regularly practice this asana. In the yoga lexicon, the Headstand is known as the "King of Asanas."

Technique:

1. Place your child on her back.

2. Sit or kneel close to your child's head.

3. Reach out over her body and grasp her lower legs just above the ankles.

4. Lift her legs off the floor.

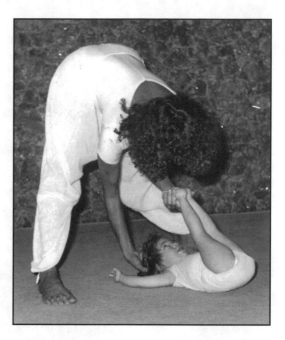

5. Continue to lift, slowly bringing her body into vertical alignment, with the top of her head lightly touching the floor. Try to keep the head in contact with the floor — this will provide a reference point to help her feel more secure.

6. Your child should now be completely upside down and facing you. Observe her face to see if she is comfortable and content to be in an inverted position. If you notice the slightest degree of discomfort, immediately bring her out of the pose.

7. Begin by holding the Headstand for 5 seconds and gradually work up to a maximum of one minute.

8. To bring her out of the pose, hold both legs with one of your hands and place your other hand at the back of her neck. Gently move her head toward you as you lower her legs.

Variation: Depending on the size of the child, you may find it easier to stand while assisting her in performing this pose (see photo at right).

 Note:

(1) It is important to allow your child to rest on her back for at least one minute after performing the Headstand so that the blood pressure can equalize throughout her body. If you raise her head too soon, it may cause her to become faint.

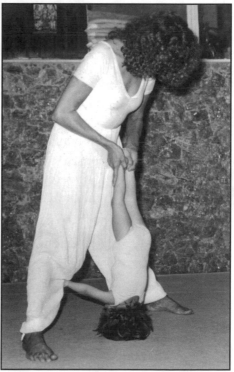

Conclusion to the Yoga Session

Exercise 26 | *Deep Relaxation*

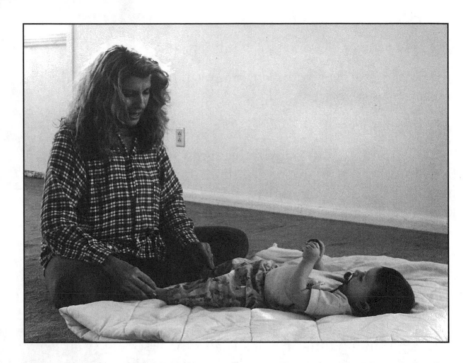

Benefits: Approximately 30 minutes have passed since the beginning of the yoga session, during which your child has had many areas of her body stretched and toned. Now it is time for her to rest, in order to assimilate the benefits of all these movements and postures. In yoga, this is accomplished through Deep Relaxation. During Deep Relaxation, as muscles and nerves release stored-up tension, a sense of calm and focus is restored. The nervous system is strengthened and general health improves. For this reason, I recommend that you always include Deep Relaxation as an integral part of your child's yoga routine.

Technique:

During Deep Relaxation your child should be kept as comfortable and still as possible. Try not to make any sudden movements that might distract her attention from the interior process that is taking place. If you wish to speak, do so quietly and in a soothing tone of voice.

Having just completed the Headstand, your child should now be resting on her back. Prepare the room by dimming the lights and putting on a cassette or CD of quiet, relaxing music. If the room seems cool or drafty, cover her with a blanket. Sit at her feet and place them 6–12 inches apart. Begin the relaxation process by massaging both feet at the same time. Massage the soles, using your thumbs in a gentle kneading motion. Then massage the top of each foot with your fingers. Allow her legs to remain resting on the floor while you massage her feet.

Depending on the child, you may wish to continue working on her feet throughout the entire relaxation period, or you may decide to stop massaging after a few minutes. Some children respond positively if you massage them from feet to head, naming each part of the body as you work on it. This type of verbal communication can help to develop greater body awareness. Other children prefer to be massaged on the nape of the neck, the face, or the top of the head. If the child has difficulty relaxing on the floor, you can try cradling her in your arms. Sometimes the closeness of this type of physical contact helps to induce a state of relaxation.

You should feel free to structure the relaxation period according to your own perception of your child's needs. By being positive, intuitive, affectionate, and loving, you will find the best way to help her relax. Don't worry if she falls asleep — she will continue to absorb the benefits of Deep Relaxation. After approximately 10 minutes, bring your child out of Deep Relaxation by chanting or gently touching the soles of her feet. Finish the yoga session with some words of encouragement and (if you wish) several hugs and kisses.

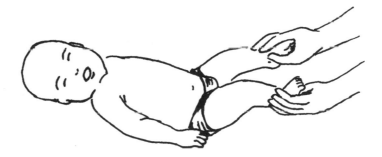

Notes and Comments on the Interactive Stage

- The Interactive Stage Program contains many more exercises than either of the previous programs. Since your child can now perform asanas more rapidly than before, she should have no difficulty completing the full routine within 40 minutes. With her newfound agility, she may even become overly enthusiastic and not want to stay in poses for the prescribed amount of time. If this happens, you should encourage her to slow down and relax. Ideally, she should remain in each pose a little longer as she becomes more adept in her practice.

- Remember to allow time in between exercises for your child to relax in preparation for the next exercise.

- In order to maintain your child's interest level, you may find it helpful to occasionally vary the sequence of her yoga routine.

- *If your child has seizures, suffers from a cardiac or spinal problem, or has had a recent illness or surgery, do not attempt to begin a program of yoga therapy without professional guidance.* You will need to contact a yoga teacher who is certified to practice the methods outlined in this book. The yoga teacher will be able to assess your child's needs and, in conjunction with your physician, prepare a yoga program that your child can safely follow.

- Developing speech and language skills requires the assistance of a speech and/or language therapist. Yoga helps to improve respiration and will complement the work of the therapist.

- Remember that your child's enthusiasm and energy level can vary from time to time. Try to be sensitive to these changes and adjust the exercises accordingly.

- Be consistent. A little yoga every day will be much more effective in the long run than a lot of yoga once in a while.

Yoga Practice Chart for the Interactive Stage

Once you have become familiar with the Interactive Stage exercises, you may use the easy-reference chart at the end of this chapter to guide you through your child's yoga routine.

Interactive Stage Exercises

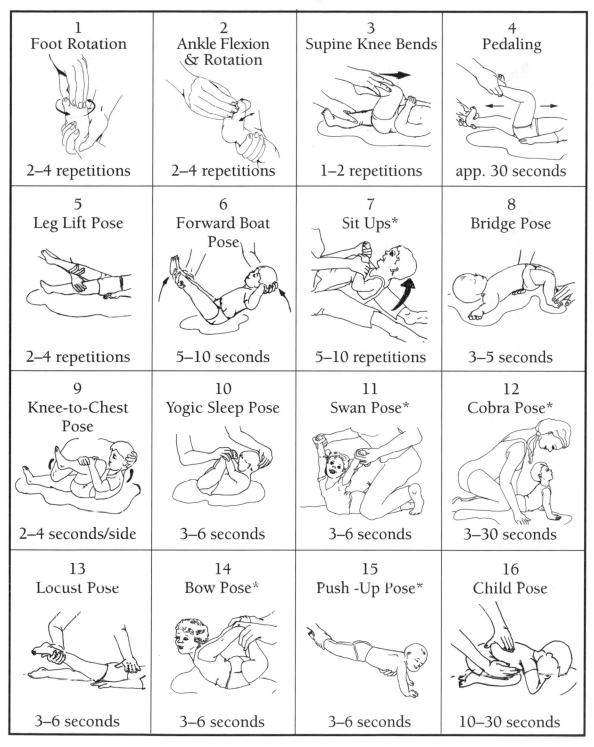

1 Foot Rotation	2 Ankle Flexion & Rotation	3 Supine Knee Bends	4 Pedaling
2–4 repetitions	2–4 repetitions	1–2 repetitions	app. 30 seconds
5 Leg Lift Pose	6 Forward Boat Pose	7 Sit Ups*	8 Bridge Pose
2–4 repetitions	5–10 seconds	5–10 repetitions	3–5 seconds
9 Knee-to-Chest Pose	10 Yogic Sleep Pose	11 Swan Pose*	12 Cobra Pose*
2–4 seconds/side	3–6 seconds	3–6 seconds	3–30 seconds
13 Locust Pose	14 Bow Pose*	15 Push-Up Pose*	16 Child Pose
3–6 seconds	3–6 seconds	3–6 seconds	10–30 seconds

Interactive Stage Exercises (Continued)

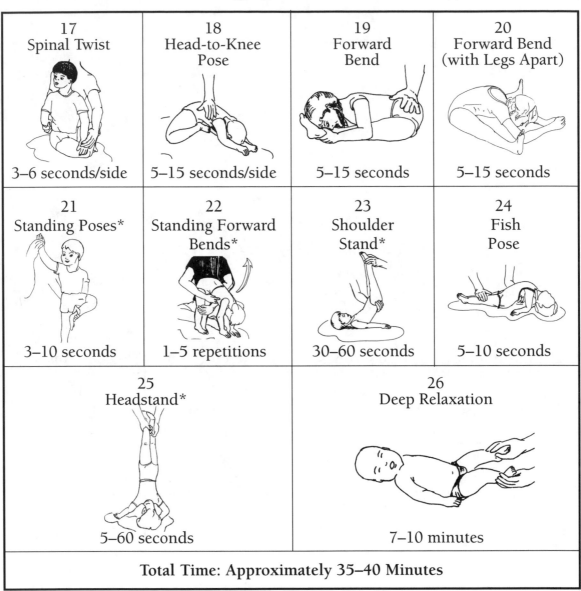

17 Spinal Twist	18 Head-to-Knee Pose	19 Forward Bend	20 Forward Bend (with Legs Apart)
3–6 seconds/side	5–15 seconds/side	5–15 seconds	5–15 seconds
21 Standing Poses*	22 Standing Forward Bends*	23 Shoulder Stand*	24 Fish Pose
3–10 seconds	1–5 repetitions	30–60 seconds	5–10 seconds
25 Headstand*		26 Deep Relaxation	
5–60 seconds		7–10 minutes	

Total Time: Approximately 35–40 Minutes

* Asterisk-marked exercises should be incorporated into your child's practice only after she has demonstrated the ability to perform them without discomfort.

8

The Imitative Stage
Developing Independence

(Two to Three Years)

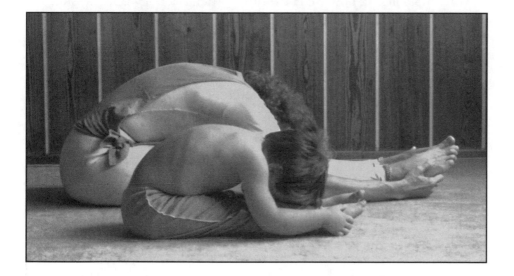

In order to begin practicing asanas in the Imitative Stage, your child needs to have mastered many basic motor and cognitive skills. He should be able to stand and walk without assistance, understand your instructions, and imitate your movements. This requires a higher level of attention and language skills than in the previous three stages, plus good body awareness, muscle tone, and flexibility. Since the child will learn most quickly by following your example, you will need to demonstrate a number of simple yoga asanas.

Introduce each new asana to your child by first performing it yourself. Clearly demonstrate and explain each movement of your body as you enter, hold, and release the pose. Show him when to inhale and exhale. In general, inhale as you raise your body or bend backward. Exhale as you lower your body or bend forward. Breathe normally while you hold a pose. Breathing properly during an asana will help the muscles to relax and make the asana much easier to perform. As a result, the body's internal rhythm, including the heartbeat and respiration, will calm down, and the benefits of the asana will be greatly enhanced. After you have demonstrated a particular pose, ask your child to repeat what you have done. Sit beside him and provide the necessary verbal instructions and physical assistance.

Once your child has mastered a particular pose, encourage him to perform it without your help, correcting his posture and providing physical assistance only when necessary. Before you correct his posture, first tell him how well he is doing; then ask if it would be okay for you to help him with a particular aspect of the pose. This type of approach will encourage him to develop greater independence and promote his cooperation throughout the yoga session. In the Imitative Stage, you will also be introducing your child to Music and Sound Therapy, Pranayama, and Eye Exercises. With the addition of these three important areas of practice, his yoga routine will have essentially the same format as our group classes for children and adults.

☑ Note: Each of the exercises in the Imitative Stage Program has been graded according to your child's ability to perform specific postures and body movements without assistance. Exercises having a greater degree of difficulty, such as inverted or standing asanas, are marked with an asterisk. It is possible that your child will need continued assistance with these asanas, as well as with the advanced variations of other asanas, until he acquires the necessary skills to perform these poses without your help.

Because you will be demonstrating poses in the Imitative Stage, the instructions provided in the asana section of this chapter are written in the second person (you). To help guide your child through a particular pose, simply repeat the instructions for that exercise in a way he can easily understand. To help him come out of the pose, repeat the same instructions in reverse order. Start with the minimum duration or number of repetitions specified for each exercise. As your child becomes accustomed to the exercises, you will be able to gradually increase these limits. Allow short rest periods between exercises as necessary.

Exercises from a Seated Position

Music and Sound Therapy

Exercise 1

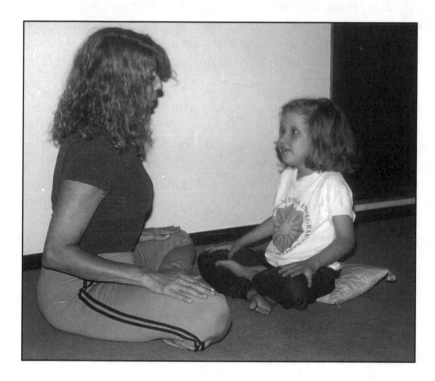

Benefits: Most children love to sing. Through the medium of song, they learn to relate to others on a personal and social level, and to express a wide range of emotions. In the case of children with disabilities, singing helps to increase their attention span and improve their memory. It also develops important skills related to voice, speech, rhythm, and motor coordination. By beginning your yoga session with 3–5 minutes of lively singing and hand clapping, you will help to create a positive and congenial atmosphere in your yoga classroom. You and your child will feel lighter, happier, and more focused during the exercises that follow.

Technique:

Sit facing your child. Adjust his shoulders and back so that he is sitting in an upright, yet relaxed position. Introduce the music session by intoning a vowel sound, such as "ah," "ē," or " ō." Once you have set the pitch, have him join in. Continue to hold the vowel sound for 5–7 seconds. Now ask him to take a deep breath. Then repeat the vowel sound a second time.

After a total of three intonations continue the music session with a short song that your child will repeat after you. The lyrics should have a positive and uplifting message. The song could be as brief as a single word like "amen" or "hallelujah." It could be a short phrase like "peace and joy" or "I see you, you see me." Depending on the child, the lyrics could be more complex. Here are some examples: "I love my mom, I love my dad, I love my dog, I love my cat;" "Peace and joy, love and light;" "Grass is green, sky is blue, you love me, and I love you." If you wish, you may also use a nursery rhyme or traditional song that your child knows.

Clap your hands together as you sing. Choose a simple melody and follow the tempo with your hand clapping. After you finish one round, wait for your child to repeat what you have sung. Help him clap his hands together until he becomes accustomed to the song's natural rhythm. When he finishes singing, repeat the round a second time and wait for his response. Continue with this responsive singing for a total of 3–5 minutes. You can vary the melody and tempo, as well as the hand clapping. Clap your hands on your knees for one or two rounds, then clap above your head for several rounds. When it comes to your child's turn, you may have to guide his hands through these new movements until he is able to imitate your hand clapping without assistance. Slow down the tempo toward the end of the music session and then sit quietly together for a few moments.

 Note: Always encourage your child to take full, deep breaths between each round. This will develop his lung capacity and teach him to coordinate speech and respiration.

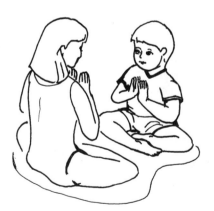

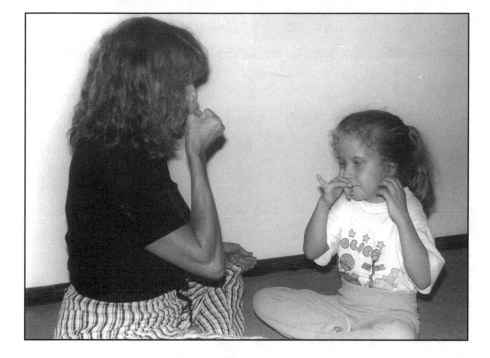

☑ **Note:** Begin the pranayama session with the Cleansing Breath. Wait until your child has mastered this exercise before including the Bellows Breath, and finally Alternate Nostril Breathing. All three exercises take a total of 5–6 minutes to perform.

The Cleansing Breath

Benefits: This pranayama removes excess mucus and phlegm from the sinuses and respiratory tract. Its powerful exhalations clear the lungs of old stale air, which is then replaced with fresh, oxygen-rich air. As a reult, the oxygen level of the blood increases, revitalizing the brain and central nervous system. The Cleansing Breath is an ideal practice for children with asthma, sinus conditions, and bronchial congestion.

Technique:

Sit facing your child. Place one or two Kleenex tissues in front of him, on his blanket. Begin with a brief explanation and demonstration of the Cleansing Breath. This exercise consists of:

1. A normal inhalation, followed by

2. A rapid exhalation. The air is expelled from the lungs by a forceful, inward-and-upward movement of the diaphragm.

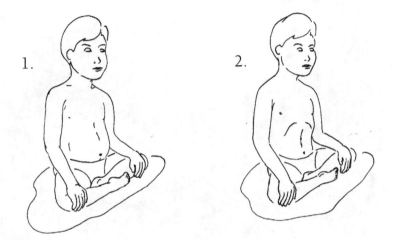

Show your child how your stomach expands on the inhalation and moves in on the exhalation. Always breathe through the nostrils, with the mouth closed. Breathing through the nostrils helps to filter and warm the air before it enters the lungs.

Now it is time for your child to perform the Cleansing Breath. Ask him to pick up a tissue and hold it in front of his nose (about 4–6 inches from his face). The tissue will help to catch any mucus that is expelled from his nose during the exhalations. Now ask him to take a deep breath and then to exhale rapidly as you count "one." Again, start with an "inhale" and then count "two" for the second exhalation. Continue until he has completed twenty inhalations and exhalations. At the end of this first set, remind him to blow his nose. Before beginning the second set, have him take 2–3 deep, slow breaths—filling the lungs and exhaling completely. Repeat the Cleansing Breath one or two more times.

 Note: Teaching your child pranayama usually requires a little extra time. The best approach is to perform this exercise in front of your child, encouraging him to join in when he feels ready. Be patient because the benefits he will reap from practicing pranayama are well worth the extra effort.

The Bellows Breath

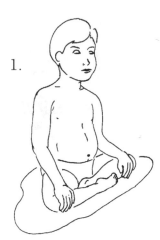

Benefits: The Bellows Breath is a highly energizing, rapid-breathing exercise, providing many of the same benefits as the Cleansing Breath. This exercise saturates the lungs and blood with freshly-oxygenated air, benefiting the entire body. The Bellows Breath's vigorous in-and-out movements of the abdomen strengthen the diaphragm, warm the body, increase circulation, and aid digestion.

Technique:

Begin with a brief explanation and demonstration of this exercise. The Bellows Breath consists of:

1. A rapid inhalation, followed immediately by

2. A rapid exhalation.

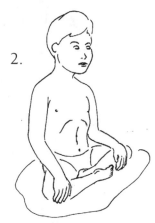

Repeat steps 1 and 2 without pausing between either the inhalations or the exhalations. Remember to breathe through the nostrils. Once again, show your child how your stomach moves in and out during this exercise. Now have your child perform the Bellows Breath until he completes a set of 20–25 inhalations and exhalations. At the end of the set, ask him to take a slow, deep breath. Do a second set and, if possible, a third.

Alternate Nostril Breathing

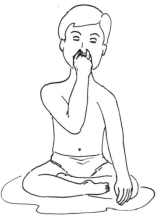

Benefits: Known as the "Nerve Purification Breath," Alternate Nostril Breathing is a wonderfully effective exercise for calming the mind. This breath strengthens the entire nervous system and helps to balance the right and left hemispheres of the brain. Among its many other benefits, Alternate Nostril Breathing strengthens the immune system, stimulates digestion, and develops concentration.

Technique:

1. You will first need to show your child how to hold his fingers during this exercise. Extend the fingers of your right hand. Bend the index and middle fingers into your palm. Keep the thumb, ring finger, and little finger extended.

2. Exhale completely.

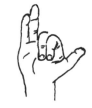

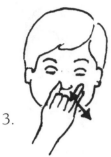

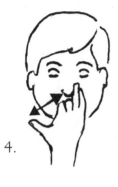

3.

4.

3. Close your right nostril with your right thumb and slowly inhale and exhale through the left nostril.

4. Remove your thumb from the right nostril and close the left nostril with your ring finger. Slowly inhale and exhale through the right nostril. This completes one round of Alternate Nostril Breathing.

When your child begins to perform Alternate Nostril Breathing, you will need to help him place his fingers in the proper position. Close off his right nostril with the thumb of his right hand. Then ask him to slowly inhale and exhale. Remove his thumb from the right nostril and close his left nostril with his ring finger. Then ask him to slowly inhale and exhale through the right nostril. Your child has now completed one round of Alternate Nostril Breathing. Continue to assist him until he has completed a total of 8–10 rounds.

Exercise 3 | *Eye Exercises*

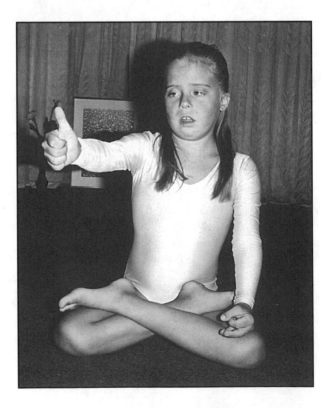

Benefits: Eye Exercises include specific movements of the eyes and the practice of focusing on near and distant objects. Eye movements tone the optic nerves and the muscles surrounding the eyes. Focusing develops visual accommodation (the automatic adjustment in the focal length of the lens of the eye). Both exercises help to improve eyesight and concentration.

Eye Movements

Technique:

1. Remain seated in front of your child. Make a fist with your hand and extend the thumb upward. Raise your arm so that your extended thumb is almost out of his field of vision. Remind him to keep his eyes focused on your thumb. Keeping the thumb extended, slowly lower your raised arm in a straight line until your hand touches the floor. This constitutes one round of up-and-down movements. Repeat several times.

2. Make horizontal movements at your child's eye level, from right to left, and back again.

3. Make diagonal movements from the upper-right to the lower-left, and back. Then make diagonal movements from the upper-left to the lower-right, and back.

4. Make two large clockwise circles in the air with your thumb. Keep your thumb at the very limit of your child's field of vision. Go slowly enough so that he can follow the movements of your thumb with his eyes. Finally, make two large circles in the opposite direction.

☑ **Note:** In place of your thumb, you can help your child to perform eye movements with a lit candle or brightly-colored object. A favorite toy or a noise-making toy, such as a squeaky rubber mouse, can also help to attract and hold his attention. As your child becomes accustomed to this exercise, you can teach him how to perform the movements with his own arm and extended thumb. This will help him to develop greater eye-hand coordination.

Focusing

❎ **Caution**: Focusing is an advanced exercise and should not be attempted until your child is comfortable performing the eye movements. Do not attempt this exercise if your child has a tendency to cross his eyes.

Technique:

Make a fist with your hand and extend your thumb upward. Hold your thumb level with your child's eyes, approximately two feet in front of him. Ask him to watch your thumb as you slowly move it toward him by extending your arm. Continue the movement until your thumb finally touches the tip of his nose. Remind him to keep looking at your thumb, even though he is now cross-eyed. Hold this position for one or two seconds, and then slowly move your thumb back to its original position.

☑ **Note:** As your child becomes accustomed to this exercise, you can teach him how to perform the movements with his own arm and extended thumb. This will help him to develop greater eye-hand coordination.

The Spinal Twist | Exercise 4

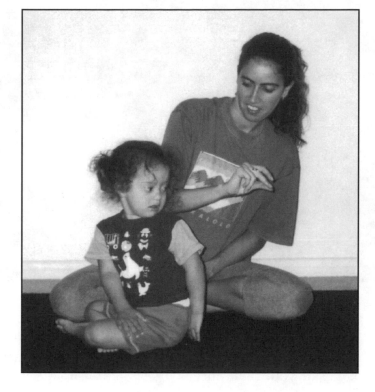

Benefits: The twisting movements of this asana stretch the connecting ligaments of the vertebrae, reduce disk compression, and stimulate nerves and ganglia in the area surrounding the spine. By compressing first one side of the body and then the other, the Spinal Twist massages and tones internal organs and glands, benefiting the liver, spleen, pancreas, kidneys, and adrenals. It also helps to relieve muscular tension in the back, waist, and hips.

Technique:

1. Sit in a comfortable cross-legged position with your spine in alignment.

2. Place your right hand on your left knee. Place your left arm behind your back. Inhale.

3. Exhale and twist your body to the left. Now twist a little more and look over your left shoulder.

4. Hold the pose for 5–15 seconds and release.

5. Face forward and repeat the Spinal Twist to the right.

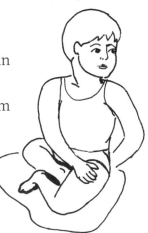

Advanced Variation:

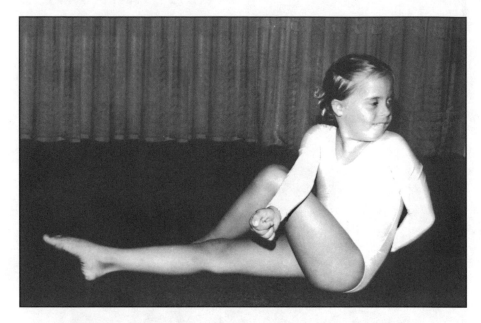

1. Extend your right leg.

2. Bend your left leg and lift it off the floor. Cross your left foot over the extended right leg and place the sole of the foot firmly on the floor, beside your right knee.

3. Gently twist your trunk to the left and place your right arm on the outside of your left knee. If possible, take hold of your right knee with your right hand. Place your left hand on the floor behind your back.

4. Straighten your back and inhale. Exhale and twist to the left. Look over your left shoulder.

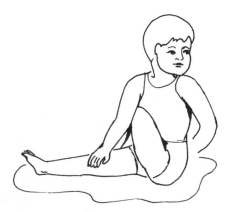

5. Breathe normally while you hold the pose for 5–15 seconds. Release the pose.

6. Face forward and repeat the Spinal Twist to the right.

The Yogic Seal | Exercise 5

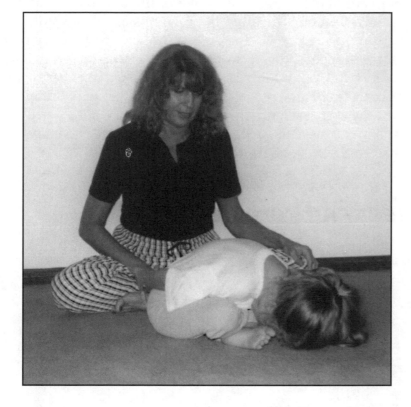

Benefits: One of the most relaxing poses, the Yogic Seal strengthens the nervous system and helps to release tension in the back muscles and spinal column. It also aids digestion and helps to prevent constipation.

Technique:

1. Sit in a comfortable, cross-legged position.

2. Put your hands behind your back and interlace your fingers.

3. Lean forward and lower your head to the floor. Keep your hands clasped behind your back.

5. Relax and breathe normally while you hold the pose for 10–20 seconds.

Forward-Bending Poses

Forward-bending poses form one of the four basic groups of asanas for the spine. The other three groups are backward-bending, twisting, and side-bending poses. The forward-bending poses reverse the stretch of the backward-bending poses; a left twist reverses the stretch of a right twist, and so on. Taken together, all four groups constitute a total program for keeping the spinal column flexible, healthy, and resilient. These complementary poses fortify the central nervous system, strengthen and elongate all the muscles of the torso, and benefit all the internal organs.

Exercise

6

The Head-to-Knee Pose

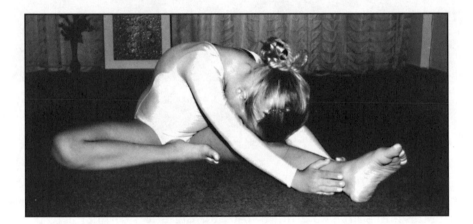

Benefits: Regular practice of the Head-to-Knee Pose helps to release tension in the lower back and to prevent constipation. It is an excellent preparation for the Forward Bend.

Technique:

1. Extend your right leg.

2. Keeping your left leg on the floor, bend the left knee and place the sole of your left foot against the inside of your right thigh. Move your left heel in toward your perineum.

3. Raise your arms above your head and stretch upward, inhaling. Exhale and bend forward from the waist. Grasp your right ankle bend forward as far as possible. Try to touch your head to your knee.

4. Hold the pose for 15–30 seconds and release.

5. Repeat the Head-to-Knee Pose with your other leg.

 Note:

(1) Allow your neck and shoulders to relax while holding the pose.

(2) Try to keep the knee of your extended leg from lifting off the floor.

The Forward Bend | *Exercise* 7

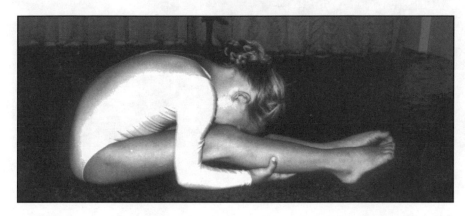

Benefits: The Foward Bend helps to elongate the spinal column by stretching the muscles and ligaments attached to the vertebrae. It gives an excellent stretch to all the posterior muscles. This asana benefits the entire body, especially the central nervous system. It tones the organs of the abdomen and helps to relieve tension in the lower back.

Technique:

1. Extend both legs in front of you. Keep your legs together and sit up straight.

2. Raise your arms overhead and stretch upward, inhaling. Bend forward from the waist, exhaling, and grasp your lower legs, ankles, or feet.

4. Hold the pose for 15–30 seconds and release.

 Note:

(1) Allow your neck and shoulders to relax while holding the pose.
(2) Try to keep your knees from lifting off the floor.

Exercise 8

The Forward Bend
(With Legs Apart)

Benefits: This asana increases range of movement in the hips and elongates the hamstrings and tendons of the inner thighs. The two variations described below are normally performed together.

Variation 1:

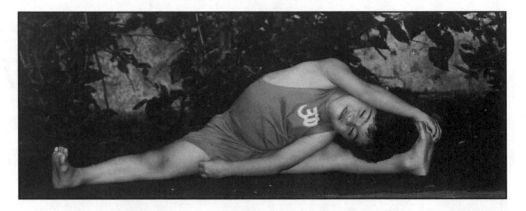

1. Extend your legs and spread them as far apart as possible. Sit up straight.

2. Raise your arms overhead and stretch upward, inhaling. Twist your trunk to the left and bend forward from the waist, exhaling. Reach out and grasp your lower leg, ankle, or foot.

3. Allow your neck to relax and hold the pose for 10–20 seconds.

4. To release the pose, return to an upright position, keeping your hands on the floor.

5. Face forward and repeat the pose with your right leg.

☑ **Note:** Keep both hips on the floor during this pose and try to resist the tendency to raise your opposite thigh off the floor when bending to one side.

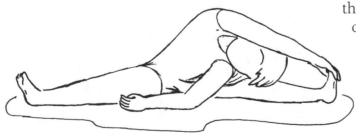

Variation 2:

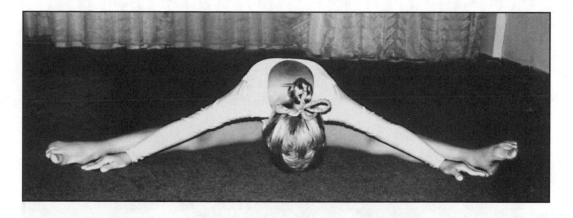

1. Keep your legs apart as you return to an upright position. Face forward and inhale.

2. Bend forward from the waist, exhaling, and lower your chest toward the floor. You can place your hands on the floor in front of you to support your body as you gradually lower down. Try to keep your back as straight as possible.

3. Hold the pose for 15–25 seconds.

☑ **Note:** If you are able to reach the floor with your forehead or chest, you can spread your arms apart and place your hands on your ankles.

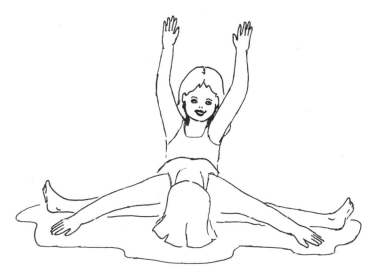

Exercises from a Supine[1] Position

Exercise 9 | *The Knee-to-Chest Pose*

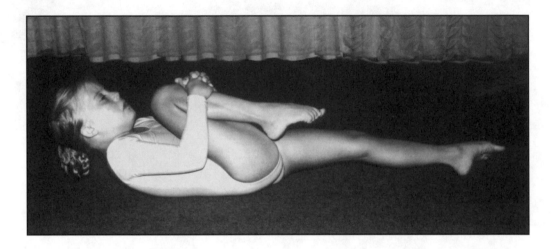

Benefits: This asana is excellent for relieving gas, colic, and other intestinal problems. It strengthens the muscles of the abdomen, stretches muscles of the back and neck, and helps to increase flexibility in the hips and knees. It is especially beneficial for relieving stress in the lower back.

Technique:

1. Lie flat on your back, with your legs straight.

2. Inhaling, slowly raise your right leg to a 45-degree angle from the floor.

3. Exhaling, bend your leg at the knee and wrap both arms around the shin. Bring your knee in toward your chest as you raise your forehead toward your knee.

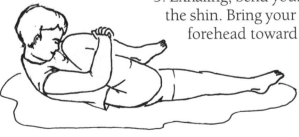

5. Hold the pose for 5–15 seconds and release.

6. Repeat with the other leg. Then repeat with both legs at the same time.

---

[1] Supine: lying on the back.

The Yogic Sleep | Exercise 10

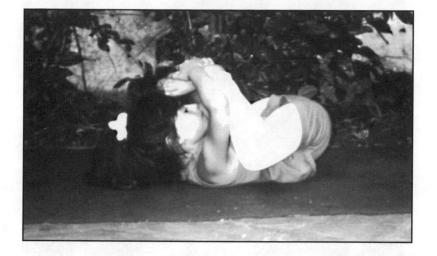

Benefits: This pose creates a forward-bending stretch along the entire spine. It also tones the organs of the abdomen and helps to increase flexibility in the hips and knees.

Technique:

1. Raise both legs to a 90-degree angle.

2. Bend your knees so that you can place both soles of your feet together.

3. Reach through the opening between your legs and grasp the outside of your feet with both hands.

4. Pull your feet toward the top of your head and raise your head toward your feet.

5. Hold the pose for 5–15 seconds.

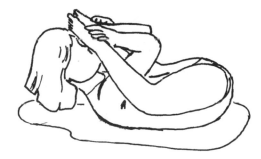

Exercise 11 | *Roll-Asana*

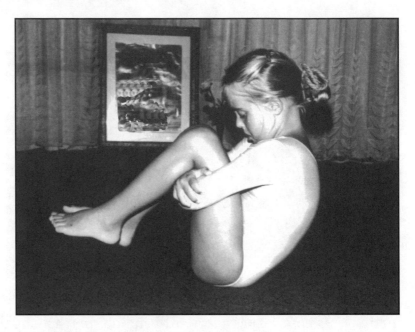

❌ **Caution:** Because Roll-Asana flexes the cervical vertebrae, it should not be performed by children with atlanto-axial instability.[2] This orthopedic problem affects 10–20 percent of children with Down Syndrome. Check with your pediatrician to make sure that your child does not have this condition.

Benefits: Children love to perform Roll-Asana. Its gentle rolling movements help to reduce compression in the spine, to release muscular tension in the back, and to tone the central nervous system.

Technique:

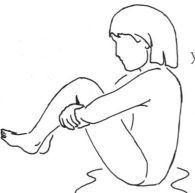

1. Lie on your back with your legs together.

2. Bend your legs at the knees and wrap your arms around your thighs. Grasp your wrist with the other hand or, if you prefer, hold onto the back of each thigh.

3. Rock backward onto your upper back. Then rock forward into a seated position, with the soles of your feet touching the floor. You can do this by extending your legs (to roll backward) and then bending them at the knees (to rock forward). Rock backward and forward, alternating the leg movements to gain momentum.

---

[2] Atlanto-axial instability is a condition of increased mobility in the joint between the atlas and the axis, the two cervical vertebrae at the base of the skull.

4. Continue rocking for 20–30 seconds. Finish this exercise by rocking up into a seated position.

Advanced Variation: Once you become accustomed to performing Roll-Asana, you can increase your range of motion by rocking backward until your feet are touching the floor behind your head.

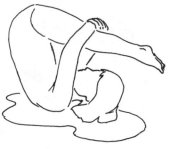

The Seated Child Pose | *Exercise* 12

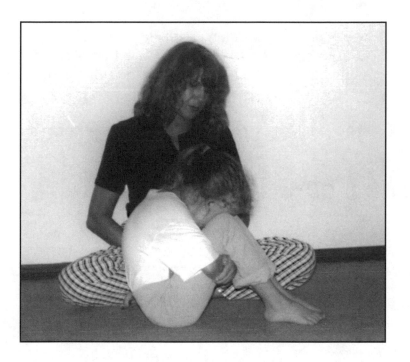

Benefits: This restful pose makes an ideal complement to the rapid movements of Roll-Asana.

Technique:

1. Remain seated with your knees bent and the soles of your feet flat on the floor.

2. Wrap your arms around your lower legs and pull your knees in toward your chest. Keep the knees together and your heels close to your buttocks.

3. Bend your head forward until it touches your knees.

4. Relax and hold the pose for 5–15 seconds.

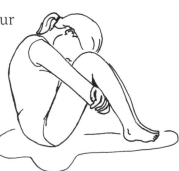

Exercises from a Prone[3] Position

 Note: Before beginning this part of the yoga session, it is a good idea to rest briefly in the following relaxation pose:

1. Lie face down with your legs comfortably apart.

2. Turn your head to one side and place your arms about 6–12 inches away from your body, with your palms facing upward.

3. Relax in this pose for 10–15 seconds.

You may do this relaxation pose before each of the backward-bending asanas. To prevent neck strain, turn your head in the opposite direction each time you perform this pose.

Backward-Bending Poses

Exercise
13

The Cobra Pose

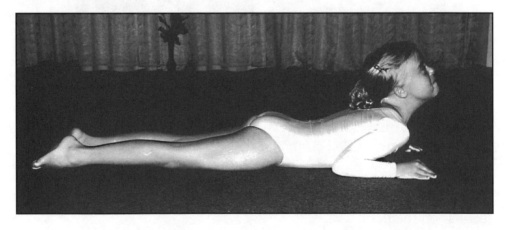

 Caution: Do not perform the advanced variations of this exercise if your child has lordosis or any other type of lower back problem.

---

[3] Prone: lying with the front or face downward.

Benefits: This asana elongates the body's anterior muscles and helps to release tension from the solar plexus and lower back. It expands the rib cage, tones the heart, lungs, and cranial nerves, and strengthens the upper back and neck muscles. It also helps to correct spinal misalignment and to relieve constipation and gas. Proceed with Advanced Variation 2 only after you have mastered Advanced Variation 1.

Technique:

1. Remain in a prone position. Bring your legs together and place your palms on the floor under your shoulders, with your fingers pointing forward.

2. Extend your neck and head so that your chin is resting on the floor.

3. Inhale and raise your upper body off the floor, beginning with your head and following with your shoulders and chest. You can accomplish this movement by extending your arms. Do not straighten your arms completely.

4. Hold the pose for 5–20 seconds.

☑ **Note:** Keep your hips on the floor throughout this exercise.

Advanced Variation 1:

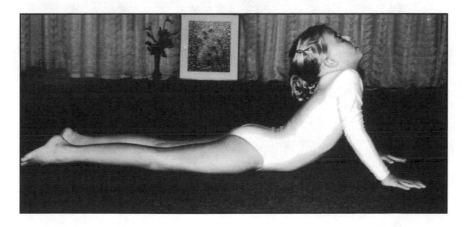

1. Perform the Cobra Pose as described above.

2. Extend your arms completely as you raise your upper body off the floor.

3. Hold the pose for 5–20 seconds.

Note: Keep your hips on the floor throughout this exercise.

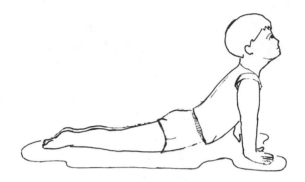

Advanced Variation 2:

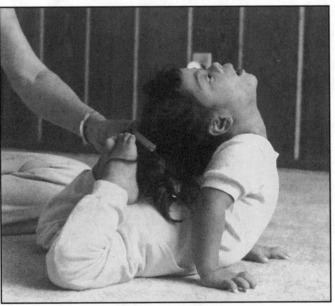

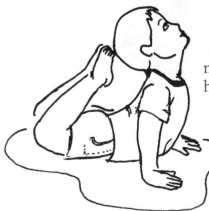

1. Perform the Cobra Pose as described in Variation 1.

2. Bend both legs at the knees. Continue this movement until the soles of your feet touch the back of your head.

3. Hold the pose for 5–20 seconds.

The Locust Pose*

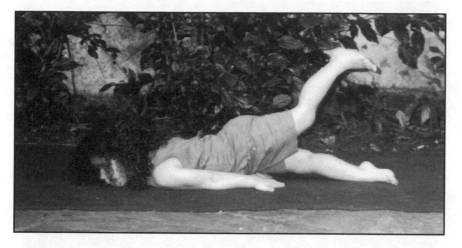

Benefits: This asana strengthens the muscles of the lower back and buttocks, stretches the abdominal muscles, and tones the organs and glands of the abdomen.

The Half Locust Pose

1. Bring your legs together and place your arms alongside your body with the palms down.

2. Tuck both arms under your body, placing your hands flat on the floor beneath your thighs.

3. Extend your neck and head so that your chin is resting on the floor.

4. Inhale and raise your left leg off the floor. Keep the leg as straight as possible. Make sure your chin and hips stay on the floor.

5. Hold the pose for 5–10 seconds and release.

6. Repeat with your right leg.

The Full Locust Pose

1. Repeat steps 1–3 of the Locust Pose.

2. Inhale and raise both legs off the floor. Keep the legs as straight as possible.

3. Hold the pose for 3–6 seconds.

*Your child may need continued assistance with asterisk-marked exercises until he is able to perform them without help.

Advanced Variation:

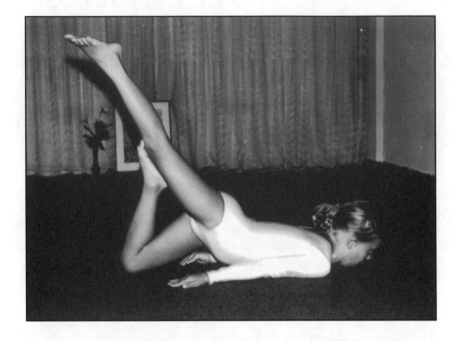

1. Assume the Locust Pose, with your right leg raised off the floor.

2. Raise the right leg a little further. Bend the left leg at the knee and place the sole of the left foot beneath your right knee.

3. Hold the pose for 5–10 seconds and release.

4. Repeat with your other leg.

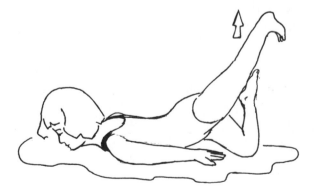

The Bow Pose* | Exercise 15

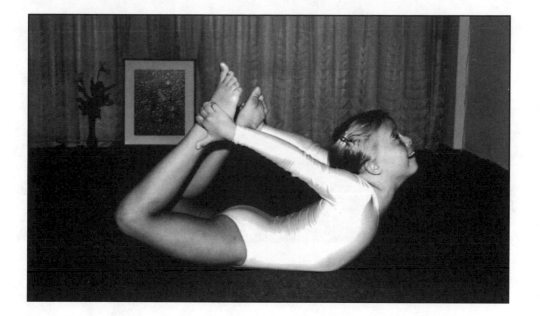

Caution: Do not perform this exercise if your child has lordosis or any other type of lower back problem.

Benefits: This asana elongates the thigh muscles and amplifies all the benefits of both the Cobra and Locust Poses. In addition, the Bow Pose reduces abdominal fat, stimulates the pancreas, and increases peristalsis in the large intestine.

Technique:

1. Bend both legs at the knees and place your forehead on the floor.

2. Grasp your ankles. Inhaling, arch your back and raise your head, chest, and thighs off the floor.

3. Hold the pose for 5–20 seconds.

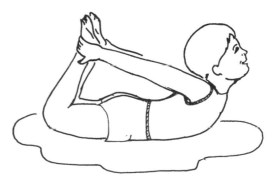

<table>
<tr><td>*Exercise*
16</td><td># The Child Pose</td></tr>
</table>

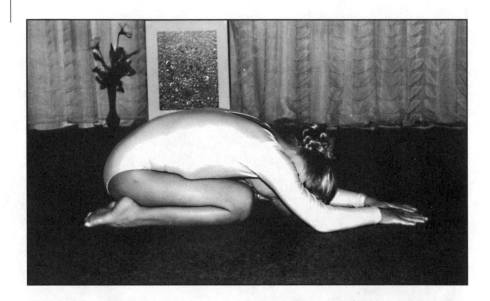

Benefits: Although technically not a backward-bending asana, the Child Pose is included in this section because it makes an excellent counter pose to the previous three exercises. This asana creates a gentle forward-bending stretch that helps to elongate the spine and reduce disk compression, especially in the lower back. Like the Knee-to-Chest Pose, it helps to relieve colic, gas, and other intestinal problems.

Technique:

1. From the prone position, come up onto your hands and knees.

2. Sit back on your heels. Slowly lower your chest down onto your thighs, and your forehead down to the floor.

3. Place your forearms and hands on the floor, either in front of you or alongside your body. Use whichever position you find more comfortable.

4. Relax and hold the pose for 10–15 seconds.

5. To release the Child Pose, raise your upper body until you are sitting up, with your feet tucked under you.

Exercises from a Standing Position

The Standing Forward Bend

Exercise

17

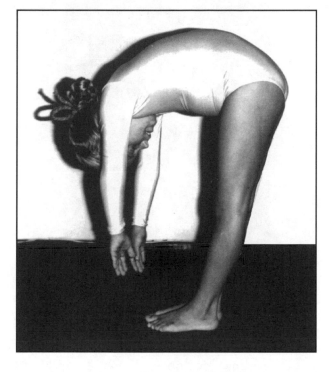

Benefits: Similar to the Forward Bend (Exercise 7), this asana uses the force of gravity to stretch the posterior muscles of the body and elongate the spinal column. It brings a fresh supply of blood to the head and tones the central nervous system. It also helps to relieve tension in the neck, shoulders, and back.

Technique:

1. Sit with your legs folded under you and your buttocks resting on your heels. Place your hands on the floor on either side of your legs.

2. Curl your toes beneath your feet.

3. Keeping both hands on the floor for support, straighten your legs. As your legs straighten, allow the force of gravity to pull your head and arms downward.

4. Hold the pose for 10–15 seconds. Keep your trunk, neck, and head relaxed during this time.

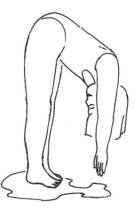

Exercise 18

*The Standing Knee-to-Chest Pose**

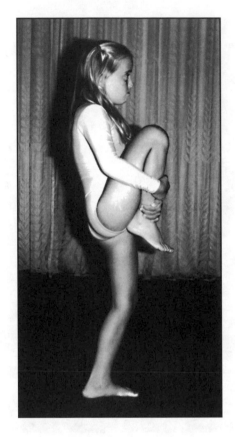

Benefits: This asana develops upper-body and leg strength and improves balance and concentration.

Technique:

1. Stand up straight with your feet together. Bring your palms together in front of your chest. Relax and feel the weight of your body distributed evenly on both feet.

2. Lower your hands and raise your right foot off the floor, bending your leg at the knee.

3. Clasp your hands or arms around your right knee and pull the knee in toward your chest.

4. Maintain your balance and hold the pose for 5–15 seconds.

5. Repeat with the other leg.

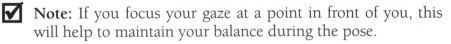 **Note:** If you focus your gaze at a point in front of you, this will help to maintain your balance during the pose.

The Triangle Pose* | *Exercise* **19**

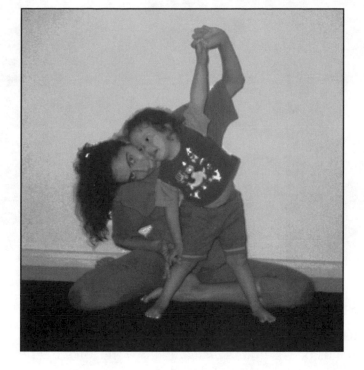

Benefits: The Triangle Pose stretches and tones the dorsal-lateral muscles, situated on either side of the spine. It improves flexibility in the spine and hips, stretches and strengthens the legs, and helps to diminish abdominal fat. This pose also tones the digestive organs, central nervous system, and adrenal glands. Once you are comfortable with the Triangle Pose, you may include the advanced variation.

Technique:

1. Stand with your legs 1–3 feet apart.

2. Inhale and raise your arms out to each side.

3. Exhale and bend your trunk to the right. Reach down your right leg with your right hand. Keep your legs straight during this movement.

4. Hold the pose for 5–15 seconds.

5. Release and repeat the Triangle Pose to the left.

 Note: This is a lateral bending pose, not a twisting pose. Try to keep your body facing forward throughout the asana.

Advanced Variation :

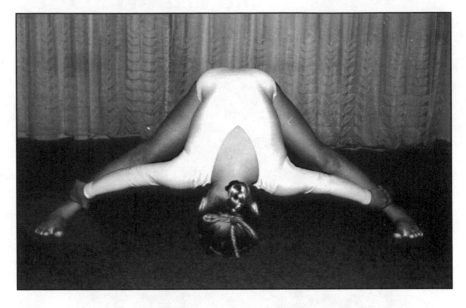

1. Repeat steps 1 and 2 of the Triangle Pose.

2. Keeping the legs straight, bend forward at the waist and place your hands on the floor. Relax and allow the force of gravity to pull your upper body and head down toward the floor

3. Hold the pose for 5–10 seconds.

☑ **Note:** The goal in performing this advanced variation of the Triangle Pose is to touch the top of your head to the floor. To increase the stretch in this pose, grasp your ankles and pull your trunk down toward the floor. Remember to keep your legs straight during this exercise and to relax the muscles of your back, neck, and head.

The Sun Salutation* | Exercise 20

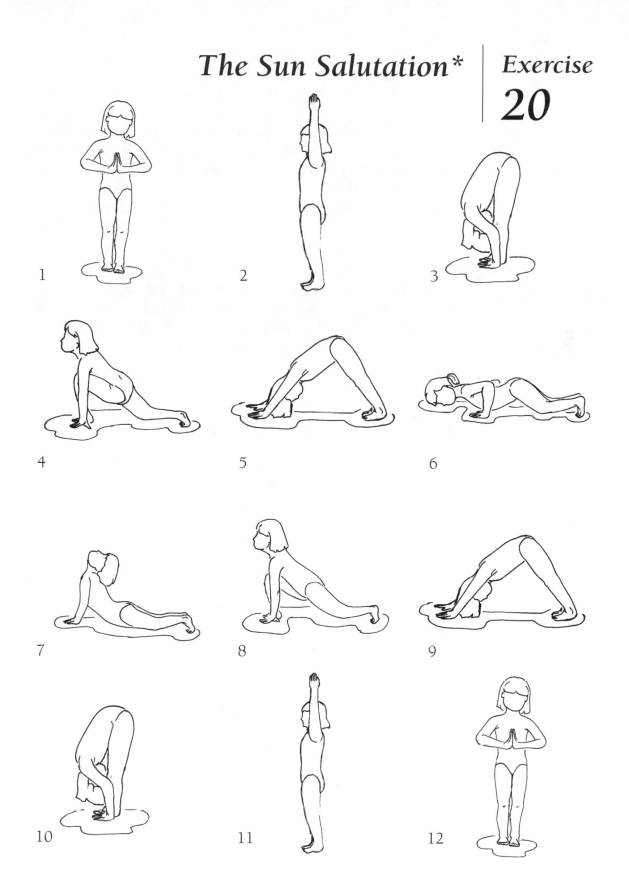

1 2 3

4 5 6

7 8 9

10 11 12

Benefits: Traditionally, the Sun Salutation is practiced early in the morning as the sun rises. It can be practiced by thyself, as an abbreviated yoga routine, or together with other asanas during your daily yoga session. The exercise consists of twelve asanas arranged in a graceful and flowing sequence. Each of these twelve poses stretches and tones a specific part of the body. Each successive pose expands or contracts the chest in a pattern of alternating inhalations and exhalations. Salutation to the Sun is a general tonic for the nervous system. It increases flexibility and lung capacity, alleviates digestive problems, and strengthens all the muscles of the body.

☑ **Note:** Wait until you are accustomed to performing the Sun Salutation before you include the instructions on respiration. Be careful not to overexert yourself during this exercise. Feel free to vary the speed and number of repetitions according to your stamina and energy level.

Technique:

Position 1

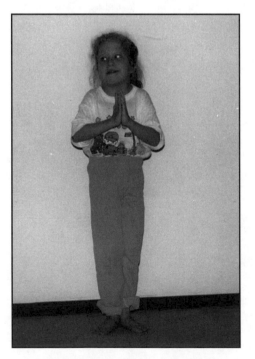

Begin in an upright, standing posture with the feet together and the palms pressed gently together in front of the chest. Exhale.

Position 2

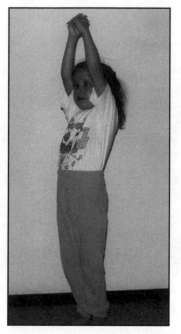

Inhaling, straighten your arms and raise them above your head. Keep your hands together and your arms in line with your ears. Stretch up.

 Caution: To avoid injury, do not allow your child to bend backward in Position 2.

Position 3

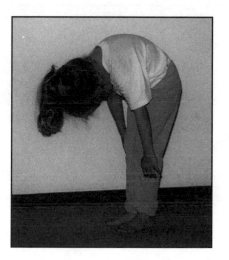

Exhaling, bend forward at the waist. Keep your legs straight and your extended arms in line with your ears as you bring your hands down toward the floor. Place your palms on the floor beside your feet.

☑ **Note:** In the beginning, you may need to bend your knees to place your palms on the floor. Keep your trunk, neck, and head relaxed while holding this pose.

Position 4

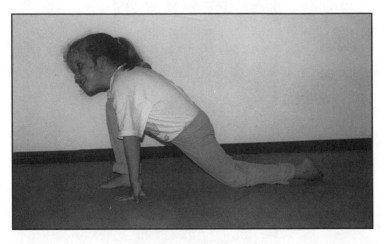

Inhaling, bend your right knee and extend your left leg backward, placing the toes and ball of your left foot on the floor. Bend your left knee so that it rests on the floor. Your right foot should be between your hands, with the right knee touching your chest. Raise your head and look up.

Position 5

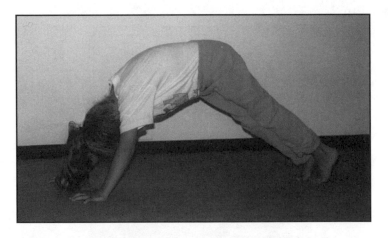

Exhaling, bring your right leg back so that it is even with the left. Straighten both legs and arms so that your body forms an inverted "V." Look back at your feet.

 Note: For an added stretch, gently press your heels to the floor while in this position.

Position 6

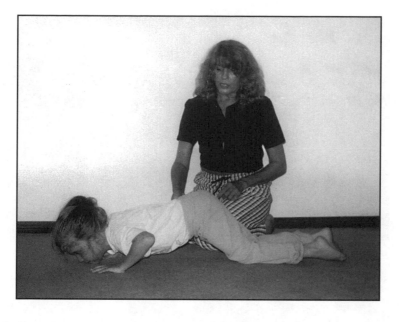

Inhaling, lower your knees to the floor. Exhaling, lower your chest and chin to the floor. Keep the hips raised several inches off the floor.

Position 7

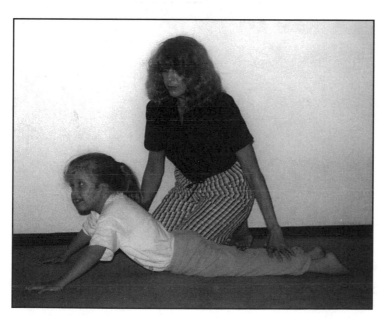

Inhaling, lower your hips to the floor. Position your palms on the floor beneath your shoulders and push up into the Cobra Pose. Do not straighten your elbows completely.

Position 8

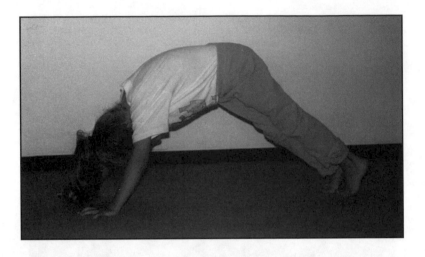

Exhaling, raise your hips up into the inverted "V" position (same as Position 5).

Position 9

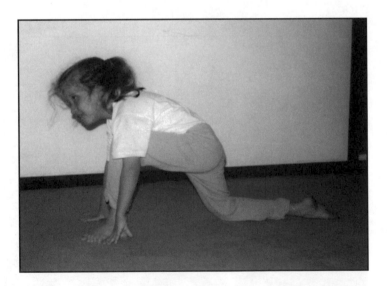

Inhaling, bend your left knee and bring the left leg forward, placing the left foot on the floor between the hands. The right leg remains extended behind your body. Bend your right knee so that it rests on the floor and lower your chest until it touches the left knee. Raise your head and look up.

Position 10

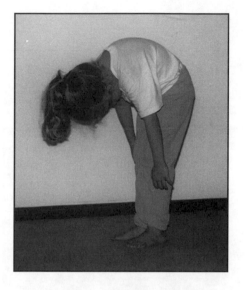

Exhaling, bring your right foot forward and place it next to the left foot. Straighten both legs. Relax and allow your head and arms to hang down toward the floor.

Position 11

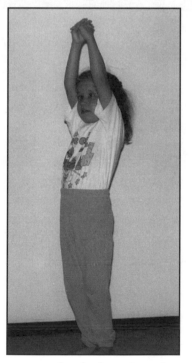

Inhaling, raise your upper body, keeping the arms alongside the ears. Stretch up (same as Position 2).

 Caution: To avoid injury, do not allow your child to bend backward in Position 11.

Position 12

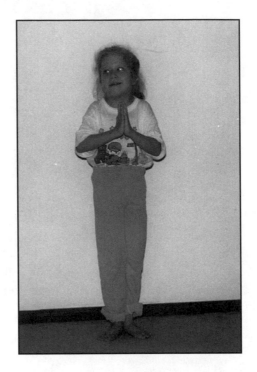

Exhaling, lower your hands and place the palms together in front of your chest (same as Position 1).

☑ **Note:** After you have completed one round of the Sun Salutation, place your legs 1–2 feet apart. Lower your arms to your sides and take 1 or 2 deep breaths before beginning a second round. Start with one repetition of the Sun Salutation and gradually work up to a maximum of three repetitions. At the end of your last round, stand with your legs 1–2 feet apart. Swing your arms to the right and then to the left. Relax your body as you swing and allow the momentum of your arms to twist your torso in the same direction. Continue swinging for 10–20 seconds.

Inverted Poses

☑ **Note:** Choose either the Shoulder Stand (and complementary Fish Pose) or the Headstand for your inverted pose. You may alternate these two poses from session to session.

*The Shoulder Stand** | *Exercise* **21**

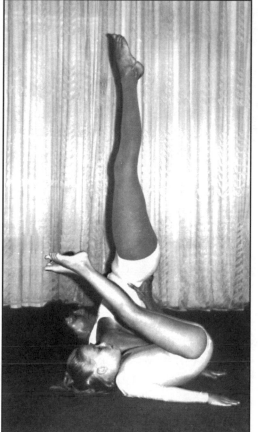

☒ **Caution:** If your child is on medication, check with your pharmacist or pediatrician to make sure that it is safe to place the child in an inverted position. If your child has a cardiac problem or seizures, then you should contact a yoga teacher who is certified to practice the methods outlined in this book. The yoga teacher will be able to assess your child's needs and, in consultation with your physician, prepare a yoga program that your child can safely follow. In addition, because the Shoulder Stand flexes the cervical vertebrae, it should not be performed by children with atlanto-axial instability.[4] Check with your pediatrician to make sure that your child does not have this condition.

Benefits: Known as the "Queen of Asanas," the Shoulder Stand is one of two inverted poses that form an integral part of almost every yoga routine. Like the Headstand, the Shoulder Stand reverses the pull of gravity and redirects the flow of blood and lymph[5] throughout the entire body. Stagnant blood is drained from the legs, and the brain and upper endocrine glands are bathed in an increased supply of fresh, oxygen-rich blood. This pose aids digestion and elimination and alleviates asthma, throat, and urinary problems. It also tones internal organs and reduces the risk of hernia and varicose veins.

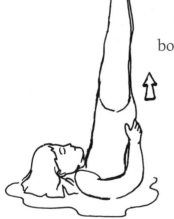

While the Headstand provides greater benefit for the pituitary and pineal glands, the Shoulder Stand concentrates its benefits in the thyroid and parathyroid glands, which regulate the body's metabolism. This asana stretches the muscles and ligaments attached to the cervical vertebrae and strengthens the muscles of the shoulders, arms, and back.

Technique:

1. Lie down on your back and place your arms alongside your body with the palms down.

2. Raise the extended legs to a 90-degree angle.

3. Using your arms for leverage, raise your entire back off the floor. Bend your arms at the elbows and place your palms against the middle of your back, on either side of the spine.

4. Using your hands to support your middle back, adjust your posture so that your entire body, from the shoulders to

---

[4] Atlanto-axial instability is a condition of increased mobility in the joint between the atlas and the axis, the two cervical vertebrae at the base of the skull.

[5] Lymph: a clear, yellowish fluid, containing white blood cells in a liquid resembling blood plasma, which is derived from the tissues of the body and conveyed to the blood stream by the lymphatic vessels.

the feet, is in a straight line. At this point, only your head, neck, shoulders, and upper arms will be touching the floor.

5. Hold the pose for 30–60 seconds.

6. To come out of the pose, slowly lower your back to the floor. Even more slowly, lower your extended legs until they are also resting on the floor.

 Note: If you experience difficulty lowering your extended legs to the floor, you may bend your knees during this movement to make it easier to perform.

Variations: Once you are comfortable performing the Shoulder Stand, you may add several variations while holding the pose. These variations stretch and strengthen the legs, back, and neck, increase mobility in the hip joints, and improve balance and body awareness. Begin with Variation 1, and add Variations 2 and 3 as you become accustomed to performing each successive variation.

Variation 1: Leg Splits

1. From the Shoulder Stand, spread your legs apart until they form a wide "V."

2. Bring the legs back together.

3. Repeat 1–3 times.

Variation 3: Leg Lifts

1. Keeping both legs straight, lower your right leg to the floor behind your head.

2. Return the right leg to a vertical position.

3. Perform the same movement with your left leg.

4. Repeat 1–3 times.

Variation 3: The Plow Pose

1. Slowly lower your extended legs to the floor behind your head.

2. Hold for 10–15 seconds and return your legs to a vertical position.

 Note: Be careful not to strain your neck or upper back as you lower your legs down into the Plow Pose.

Exercise 22 | *The Fish Pose*

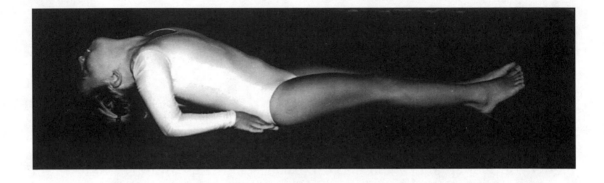

☒ **Caution:** Because the Fish Pose flexes the cervical vertebrae, it should not be performed by children with atlanto-axial instability. Check with your pediatrician to make sure that your child does not have this condition.

Benefits: This asana is the traditional counter-pose to the Shoulder Stand, opening areas of the neck and chest that were compressed in the inverted posture. Practicing the Fish Pose directly after the Shoulder Stand helps to relieve stiffness in the neck and shoulders. It complements the Shoulder Stand's benefits to the nervous system and upper endocrine glands, especially the thyroid.

Technique:

1. Bring your legs together and place your arms alongside your body.

2. Pressing down on the elbows, raise your head and back off the floor.

3. Arch your neck back until the top of the head is touching the floor.

4. Breathe deeply while you hold the pose for 10–20 seconds.

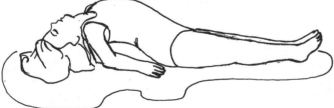

5. To release the pose, press down on the elbows, raise your head, and slowly lower your back and head to the floor.

The Headstand* | Exercise 23

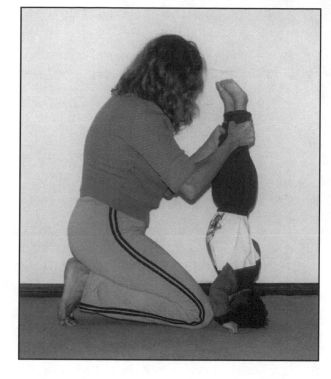

Caution: If your child is on medication, check with your pharmacist or pediatrician to make sure that it is safe to place the child in an inverted position. If your child has a cardiac problem or seizures, then you should contact a yoga teacher who is certified to practice the methods outlined in this book. The yoga teacher will be able to assess your child's needs and, in consultation with your physician, prepare a yoga program that your child can safely follow.

Benefits: By reversing the pull of gravity, the Headstand redirects the flow of blood and lymph throughout the entire body. Stagnant blood is drained from the legs, and the brain and upper endocrine glands are bathed in an increased supply of fresh, oxygen-rich blood. This pose benefits the entire nervous system, as well as the sense organs that are connected to the brain through the nerves. Scientific tests have shown that the Headstand improves memory and intellect.

This pose also aids digestion and elimination, alleviates urinary problems, tones internal organs, and reduces the risk of

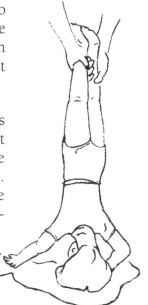

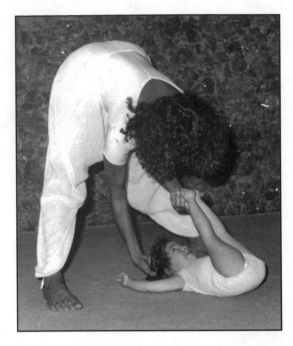

hernia and varicose veins. Because of these accumulated benefits, an overall sense of well-being is experienced by students who regularly practice this asana. In the yoga lexicon, the Headstand is known as the "King of Asanas."

Technique:

1. Place your child on his back.

2. Sit by your child's head.

3. Reach out over his body and grasp his lower legs, just above the ankles.

4. Lift his legs off the floor.

5. Continue to lift, slowly bringing his body into vertical alignment, with the top of his head lightly touching the floor. Try to keep his head in contact with the floor — this will provide a reference point to help him feel more secure.

6. Your child should now be completely upside down and facing you. Observe his face to see if he is comfortable and content to be in an inverted position. If you notice the slightest degree of discomfort, immediately bring him out of the pose.

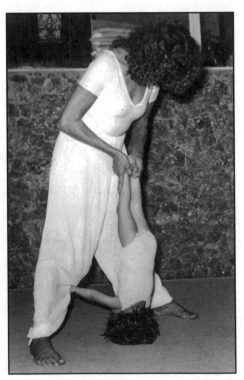

7. Begin by holding the Headstand for 5 seconds and gradually work up to a maximum of 1 minute.

8. To bring him out of the pose, hold both legs with one of your hands and place your other hand at the back of his neck. Gently move his head toward you as you lower his legs.

Variation: Depending on the size of the child, you may find it easier to stand while assisting him in performing this pose (see adjacent photograph).

☑ **Note:** It is important to allow your child to rest on his back for at least 1 minute after performing the Headstand so that the blood pressure can equalize throughout his body. If you raise his head too soon, it may cause him to become faint.

Advanced Variation:

☒ **Caution:** Because the Advanced Variation of the Headstand places pressure on the cervical vertebrae, it should not be performed by children with atlanto-axial instability. Before beginning this exercise, check with your pediatrician to make sure that your child does not have this condition. For additional precautions, read the beginning of this exercise.

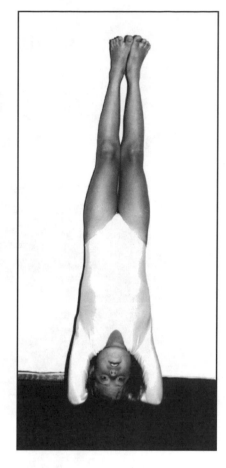

1. Sit facing a wall or corner that is free of furniture. Adjust your posture so that your legs are folded under you and your knees are 1–2 feet from the wall.

2. Place your forearms on the floor with your hands 6–12 inches from the wall. Interlace your fingers and spread your elbows shoulder-width apart.

3. Place the top of your head on the floor and support the back of your head with your palms.

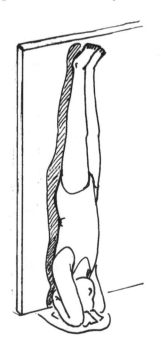

4. Straighten your legs enough to bring your torso into a vertical position.

5. Very slowly, shift your weight toward the wall. As you do so, your feet will naturally lift off the floor.

6. Little by little, raise your legs until your entire body is perpendicular to the floor and your heels are resting against the wall.

7. Hold the pose for 5–20 seconds.

8. To come out of the pose, slowly lower your legs to the floor.

9. Relax in the Child Pose for 10–20 seconds.

Conclusion to the Yoga Session

**Exercise
24** | *Deep Relaxation*

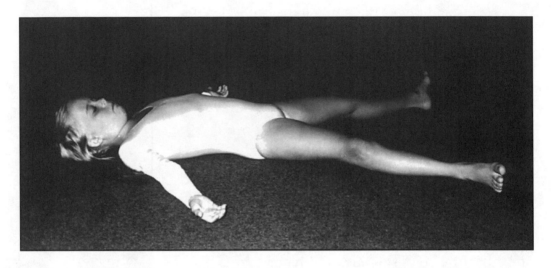

Benefits: Approximately 30 minutes have passed since the beginning of the yoga session, during which your child has had many areas of his body stretched and toned. Now it is time for him to rest, in order to assimilate the benefits of all these movements and postures. In yoga, this is accomplished through Deep Relaxation. During Deep Relaxation, as muscles and nerves release stored-up tension, a sense of calm and focus is restored. The nervous system is strengthened and general health improves. For this reason, I recommend that you always include Deep Relaxation as an integral part of your child's yoga routine.

Technique:

During Deep Relaxation your child should be kept as comfortable and still as possible. Try not to make any sudden movements that might distract his attention from the interior process that is taking place. If you wish to speak, do so quietly and in a soothing tone of voice.

Having just completed the Headstand, your child should now be resting on his back. Prepare the room by dimming the lights and putting on a cassette or CD of quiet, relaxing music. If the room seems cool or drafty, cover him with a blanket. Sit at his feet and place them 6–12 inches apart. Begin the relaxation process by massaging both feet at the same time. Massage the soles, using your thumbs in a gentle kneading motion. Then massage the top of each foot with your fingers. Allow his legs to remain resting on the floor while you massage his feet.

Depending on the child, you may wish to continue working on his feet throughout the entire relaxation period, or you may decide to stop massaging after a few minutes. Some children respond positively if you massage them from feet to head, naming each part of the body as you work on it. This type of verbal communication can help to develop greater body awareness. Other children prefer to be massaged on the nape of the neck, the face, or the top of the head. If the child has difficulty relaxing on the floor, you can try cradling him in your arms. Sometimes the closeness of this type of physical contact helps to induce a state of relaxation.

Feel free to structure the relaxation period according to your own perception of your child's needs. By being positive, intuitive, affectionate, and loving, you will find the best way to help him relax. Don't worry if he falls asleep—he will continue to absorb the benefits of Deep Relaxation. After approximately 10 minutes, bring your child out of Deep Relaxation by chanting or gently touching the soles of his feet. Finish the yoga session with some words of encouragement and (if you wish) several hugs and kisses.

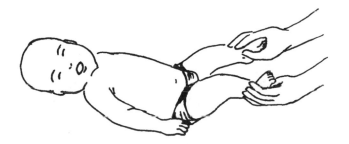

Notes and Comments on the Imitative Stage

- A complete yoga session, including Deep Relaxation, should last 35–40 minutes.

- In order to maintain your child's interest level, you may find it helpful to occasionally vary the sequence of his yoga routine.

- Your child should inhale while raising his body or bending backward and exhale while lowering his body or bending forward. He should breathe normally while holding a pose. Gently correct him when you see him breathing improperly. In time, he will learn the natural pattern for respiration.

- Remember to allow time in between exercises for your child to relax in preparation for the next exercise.

- Remember that your child's enthusiasm and energy level can vary from time to time. Try to be sensitive to these changes and adjust the exercises accordingly.

- *If your child has seizures, suffers from a cardiac or spinal problem, or has had a recent illness or surgery, do not attempt to begin a program of yoga therapy without professional guidance.* You will need to contact a yoga teacher who is certified to practice the methods outlined in this book. The yoga teacher will be able to assess your child's needs and, in consultation with your physician, prepare a yoga program that your child can safely follow.

- Developing speech and language skills requires the assistance of a speech and/or language therapist. Yoga helps to improve respiration and will complement the work of the therapist.

- Be consistent. A little yoga every day will be much more effective in the long run than a lot of yoga once in a while.

Yoga Practice Chart for the Imitative Stage

Once you have become familiar with the Imitative Stage exercises, you may use the easy-reference chart at the end of this chapter to guide you through your child's yoga routine.

Table 1. Imitative Stage Exercises

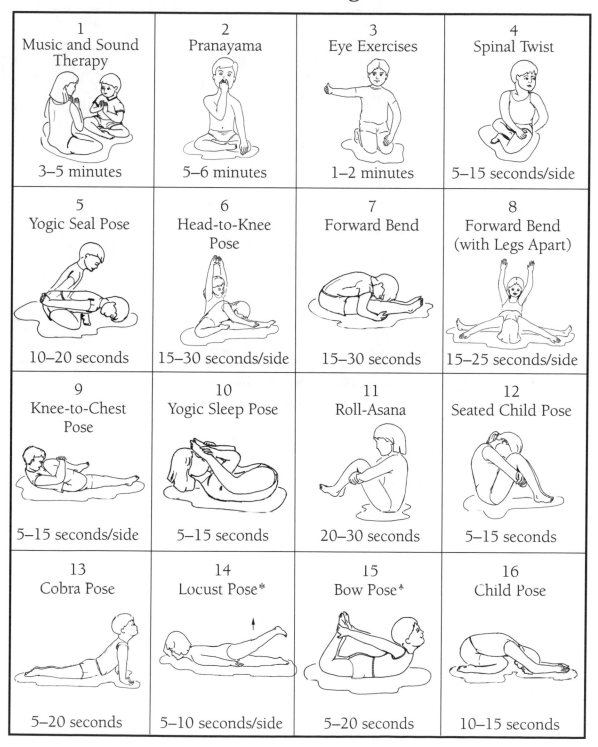

1 Music and Sound Therapy 3–5 minutes	2 Pranayama 5–6 minutes	3 Eye Exercises 1–2 minutes	4 Spinal Twist 5–15 seconds/side
5 Yogic Seal Pose 10–20 seconds	6 Head-to-Knee Pose 15–30 seconds/side	7 Forward Bend 15–30 seconds	8 Forward Bend (with Legs Apart) 15–25 seconds/side
9 Knee-to-Chest Pose 5–15 seconds/side	10 Yogic Sleep Pose 5–15 seconds	11 Roll-Asana 20–30 seconds	12 Seated Child Pose 5–15 seconds
13 Cobra Pose 5–20 seconds	14 Locust Pose* 5–10 seconds/side	15 Bow Pose* 5–20 seconds	16 Child Pose 10–15 seconds

Imitative Stage Exercises (Continued)

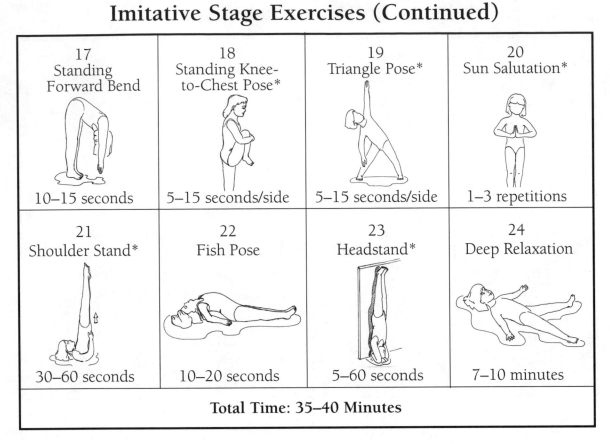

17 Standing Forward Bend	18 Standing Knee- to-Chest Pose*	19 Triangle Pose*	20 Sun Salutation*
10–15 seconds	5–15 seconds/side	5–15 seconds/side	1–3 repetitions
21 Shoulder Stand*	22 Fish Pose	23 Headstand*	24 Deep Relaxation
30–60 seconds	10–20 seconds	5–60 seconds	7–10 minutes
Total Time: 35–40 Minutes			

* Your child may need continued assistance with asterisk-marked exercises until he is able to perform them without help.

9

Teaching Group Classes
(Ages Three and Up)

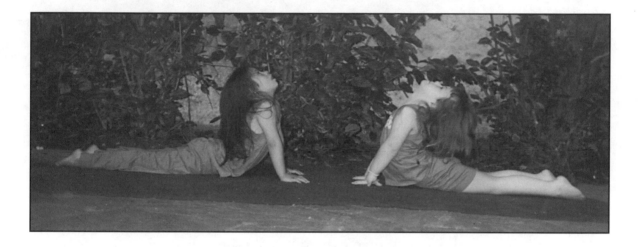

Group yoga classes provide a unique opportunity for children to develop important socialization skills. Since children enjoy interacting with each other, practicing together in a group is also an excellent way to reinforce their interest in yoga. The classes include children with various types of disabilities, as well as children without special needs. Each children's class meets twice a week and lasts approximately 45 minutes.

A typical children's class follows the same basic outline as the Imitative Stage Program. The class begins with Music and Sound Therapy, followed by Pranayama, Eye Exercises, asanas, and Deep Relaxation. Sometimes we vary the structure of the class to maintain the student's interest level. One option is to begin the class with Pranayama and to end with Music Therapy. Another possibility is to begin with Eye Exercises and to end with Pranayama and Music Therapy.

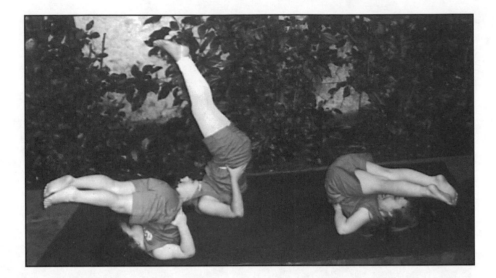

Students practicing the Shoulder Stand

The asana portion of the class consists of the following: (1) Salutation to the Sun; (2) forward-bending poses; (3) backward-bending poses; (4) twisting poses; (5) strengthening poses; (6) lateral-bending poses; (7) balancing poses; and (8) inverted poses. The teacher may vary the sequence of poses from session to session, depending on the needs of the students. However, I find it helpful to conclude the asana portion of my classes with one of the inverted poses since these poses naturally lead into Deep Relaxation. You may refer to the chart on the following page for more details on conducting a children's yoga class.

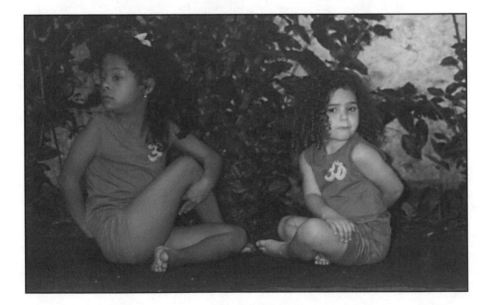

Two variations of the Spinal Twist

Children's Group Class

Area of Practice	Exercise Time	Description
Music and Sound Therapy	5 - 7 minutes	Group Chanting and Hand Clapping
Pranayama	5 - 10 minutes	Cleansing Breath, Bellows Breath, Alternate Nostril Breathing
Eye Exercises	1 - 2 minutes	Eye Movements and Focusing
Asanas:	Total Time: 20 - 25 minutes	
Sun Salutation	3 repetitions	A flowing sequence of 12 postures
Forward-Bending Poses	perform all 10 poses	Head-to-Knee Pose, Forward Bend, Forward Bend (with Legs Apart), Knee-to-Chest Pose, Yogic Sleep Pose, Roll-Asana, Yogic Seal Pose, Standing Forward Bend, Child Pose, Seated Child Pose
Backward-Bending Poses	choose 3 out of 4 poses	Cobra Pose, Locust Pose, Bow Pose, Bridge Pose
Twisting Poses	choose 1 of 2	Supine Spinal Twist, Seated Spinal Twist
Strengthening Poses	choose 1 of 3	Forward Boat Pose, Leg Lift Pose, Push-Up Pose
Lateral-Bending Poses	perform 1 pose	Triangle Pose
Balancing Poses	choose both	Tree Pose, Standing Knee-to-Chest Pose
Inverted Poses	choose 1 of 2	Headstand, Shoulder Stand (followed by Fish Pose)
Deep Relaxation	7 - 10 minutes	Deep Relaxation or Dynamic Relaxation
Total Time: 45–50 Minutes		

Note: Instructions for the above exercises can be found in Chapters 7 and 8.

I have found that children are more receptive to yoga when they enjoy the learning experience. This comes about as a natural result of the teacher's spontaneity and creativity. At the same time that you and your students are having fun, you should make every effort to maintain the keenest awareness of their individual needs and capabilities. In order to teach well, you will need to be careful, but not overly cautious; attentive, yet relaxed; and in control, but not controlling. With experience, you will be able to develop and refine the teaching style that works best for you.

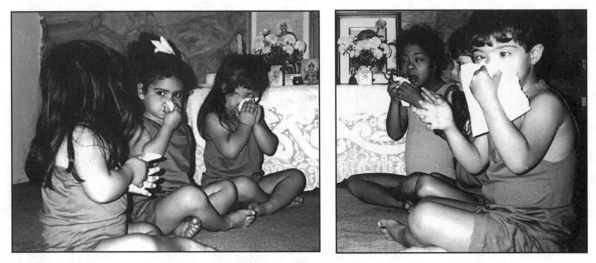

Students practicing The Cleansing Breath

Listed below are several techniques that I use in my children's yoga classes to make them more interesting and fun:

Student Teaching

Once a month, ask one of your students to lead the class. Have the child sit up front where the teacher usually sits. Stay in the back of the classroom and provide any assistance that your student teacher may need while instructing the class. As a variation, try dividing your yoga routine into several segments. Have a different student teach each segment of the class.

Dynamic Relaxation

This next practice may be occasionally substituted for the standard Deep Relaxation at the end of the yoga session. Here is an example of what you might say to your students:

Stand up and place your feet approximately two palm-widths apart. Close your eyes and be aware of your feet touching the floor. (If you wish, you may cover your students' eyes with bandanas; this will help to prevent peeking.) Bend your knees and straighten them, relaxing your legs completely. Relax your hips, stomach, chest, shoulders, and arms. Now pay attention to your breath. Gently place your hand on your chest and feel the beating of your heart. Allow your hand to return to your side and continue to focus on the beating of your heart, sensing its calm and regular rhythm. Gently roll your head, first clockwise, and then counterclockwise. Now relax your neck and face.

Keeping your eyes closed, start to walk very slowly around the room. Try to be aware of your body as you move. If you brush against another student, just be aware of the contact and keep moving. If you wish to experiment with yoga poses instead of walking, you may try practicing asanas with your eyes closed. Or, if you prefer, try dancing alone. Whatever movements you make, perform them slowly and deliberately. If you brush against another person while dancing, the two of you may try dancing together, still keeping your eyes closed.

After 5–10 minutes of this exercise, have your students quietly sit down in the same spot where they are standing. Ask them to slowly open their eyes and look around. Let each student share his or her experience of Dynamic Relaxation.

Asana Practice from Drawings

This last technique is one of the children's favorites. It may be substituted for the regular asana portion of the class and requires the use of a blackboard. Begin with a story about a young boy or girl who loves to practice yoga. My "hero" was named João Bolinha, based on a Brazilian cartoon character of the same name. João was made out of tennis balls and had a very flexible body. His greatest virtue, however, was that he was easy to draw. Whenever I described the adventures of João Bolinha, he was always performing all sorts of marvelous asanas.

Once you have told your story, ask one of your students to come up to the front of the class. Draw an asana on the blackboard and ask your student, "Do you know what asana João Bolinha is performing? Do you think you can perform this asana just like him?" Let the student perform the asana in front of the class. One by one, ask each of your students to come up and perform a different asana from your story. This technique is excellent for developing concentration and body awareness.

Notes and Comments on Teaching Group Classes

- A complete yoga session, including Deep Relaxation, should last 45–50 minutes.

- Depending on the number of your students, you may wish to divide them into two children's classes: one for ages 3–7, and the other for ages 8–12. Older students may practice in a regular adult class.

- Try to give equal time to each student. This may not be possible in all cases, but it is important that you make an effort to prevent any one student from occupying a greater share of class time than the other students.

- You may use the following general guidelines in teaching yoga to children with different types of disabilities:

    1. If a child is hypotonic, use more muscle-strengthening exercises, focusing on the areas of the body that are weakest.

    2. If a child is hypertonic, use more asanas that will elongate the areas of tightness.

    3. If a child is hyperactive or easily distracted, spend less time in each asana and more time doing Music Therapy and Pranayama. Sometimes it helps to remind the child to pay attention or to make a game out of doing the asanas. Each child is different, so you will need to develop your creativity and intuition in this type of work.

- I recommend the following minimum requirements for anyone wishing to become a professional yoga teacher of children with special needs:

    1. To successfully complete a teacher training program at an accredited yoga school.

    2. To successfully complete a Yoga for the Special Child™ Ten-Day Certification Program.

Information on Yoga for the Special Child™ Certification Programs, including a listing of program dates and locations, is available through our office at (804) 969-2668. The same information may also be found on our website at www.specialyoga.com.

In Praise of
Yoga for the Special Child

I am delighted to read the book *Yoga for the Special Child* by Sonia Sumar. Sonia has been a very dedicated and devoted yoga teacher for many years. I met her on my first trip to South America, during which time she organized a talk for me in Belo Horizonte. I visited her yoga school and saw firsthand her wonderful service to God's special children.

Children with Down Syndrome are God's children also. They are human beings also created in God's image. They may have some physical and mental limitations, but these are only challenges, not *who* they are. Essentially we are all God's children, and before God we are all loved and valued the same.

I am glad that Sonia Sumar has come forward and written a book that can give help and hope to children with Down Syndrome (and other developmental disabilities). Yoga is the master key which opens any lock. Sonia has proven this with her own daughter and now shares her wealth of knowledge and personal experience with everyone.

May God bless Sonia Sumar to continue her loving and dedicated service in the name of yoga. May the potential of each child who practices yoga expand to the fullest, and may each one know that he or she is beloved and special in the eyes of God.

Swami Satchidananda
Buckingham, Virginia
July 1994

Swami Satchidananda is a renowned teacher and ecumenical leader who has helped countless people achieve greater health and peace of mind through yoga. For close to a decade, he has been a sincere supporter of Sonia Sumar's program and teaching methods.

In her book, *Yoga for the Special Child*, Sonia Sumar shares the results of her many years of experience working with special children. An accomplished and dedicated yoga teacher, Sonia has helped many children to lead healthier, happier, and more productive lives. This is all due to her teaching methods, patience, and great love for her work. *Yoga for the Special Child* will be invaluable to parents, yoga teachers, health care professionals, and educators.

We need to remind ourselves that all children are naturally "special" in one way or another. Only by learning to love and understand them will we be able to truly assist them in developing their full potential.

Indra Devi
Buenos Aires, Argentina
December 1993

Indra Devi has been a dynamic and charismatic teacher of yoga for more than a half a century. She was one of the first Westerners to popularize Hatha Yoga in both South America and the United States. At the age of 97, she continues to offer instruction at her yoga school in Buenos Aires, Argentina.

Acknowledgments

I wish to offer my sincere gratitude to Swami Satchidananda for his guidance in the study and practice of yoga.

To my daughter, Renata, for her assistance in putting together the earlier editions of this book, I offer my heart-felt appreciation.

Special thanks go to my fiancé, Jeffrey Volk, who coordinated the translation and publication of this present English edition. Without his loving and unconditional support, this project would not have been possible.

Sonia Sumar
Belo Horizonte, Brazil
December 1997

A Note from the Coordinator of the English Translation

I would like to gratefully acknowledge the following people who contributed their time and assistance to this project: Mayapriya Long of Bookwrights Press for her assistance in preparing this book for publication; Adriana Maruso for the original translation; Helena Mader for specific translations and editing assistance; Paula Stone for editing and research; Eric Freedman for editing and consultation in the field of special education; my brother Ken Volk for editing; Prakash Capon and Renata Sumar for indexing; Shanti Wagner for the cover illustration; Renata Sumar and Roger Felicissimo for photographs; Leonardo Dinis for text illustrations; Dhyani Simonini and David Steinberg for illustration corrections; Paul Forrest, Abhaya Thiele, Lewis Randall, Swami Sarvaananda, Prem Anjali, Jnanam MacIsaac, Philip Mandelkorn, and Tom Kergel for editing assistance; and the many others who so kindly offered their time and energy.

Jeffrey Volk
Buckingham, Virginia
December 1997

We are indebted to the parents of the following children, who appeared in photographs throughout this book:

Renata Paes Bataglia

Mariana Garcia Botelho

Paula Monique Mendes Braga

Aparecida Cristina Campos

Isabela da Costa

Thomas Fionn Crombie-Angus

Arthur Arabe Lima Fonesca

Isabela Magalhães Giani

Helinho Resende Gomes

Param Johnson

Eloísa Piedade Kilson

Maurício Macagnnan

Henrique Santana Magalhães

Luiza Barroso Marques

Lorena Buval Moreira

Kaique José dos Reis Leão de Oliveira

Thaíza Ude Marques de Oliveira

Delfim Florentino Filadélfia Passos

Gabriel Rau

Henrique de Souza Ribeiro

Karina Ribeiro

Thiago Ribeiro

Luciana Sczerner da Silva

Thurston Stish

Mariana Andrade Tolentino

Glossary

Asana. Any posture or pose that can be held with steadiness and comfort.

Atlanto-axial Instability. A condition of increased mobility in the joint between the atlas and the axis, the two cervical vertebrae at the base of the skull.

Attention Deficit Disorder (ADD). It is the term used when the primary characteristic is significant inattentiveness and impulsivity, with or without hyperactivity. The child often fails to finish projects, seems not to listen, is easily distracted, and has difficulty concentrating even on a chosen task. Other thoughts, sights, or sounds keep getting in the way, especially when the task is difficult or uninteresting. The child acts before thinking, switches from activity to activity, needs a lot of supervision, and has difficulty with organization of time, work, and belongings.

Belo Horizonte. A city of three million, situated some 300 miles north of Rio de Janeiro, Brazil.

Cat's Cry Syndrome (Cri du Chat Syndrome). A genetic disorder caused by loss or misplacement of genetic material from the fifth chromosome. Named for the sound that many of the children make when crying, the syndrome causes a varied level of mental handicap.

Central Nervous System. The brain and the spinal cord. The part of the nervous system primarily involved in voluntary movement and thought processes.

Cerebral Palsy. A broad term used to describe a variety of chronic conditions in which brain damage, usually occurring at birth, impairs motor function and control.

Chromotherapy. A therapy that uses different colored lights to stimulate the body's natural healing process.

Congenital. Present at or before birth.

Cyanosis. A bluish discoloration of the skin, resulting from inadequate oxygenation of the blood.

Development. The process of growth and learning during which a child acquires skills and abilities.

Developmental Disabilities. A handicap or impairment beginning before the age of eighteen which may be expected to continue indefinitely and which causes a substantial disability. Such conditions include pervasive developmental disorders, autism, cerebral palsy, and mental retardation.

Down Syndrome. A chromosomal abnormality that results in mild to severe mental retardation and multiple birth defects. While retardation is the most familiar problem associated with Down Syndrome, affected children have a range of problems. About forty percent of all patients with Down Syndrome have heart defects. They also may have thyroid problems and intestinal abnormalities. In addition to mental retardation, they may have vision and hearing impairment and language delays. Some of the physical signs of Down Syndrome are evident soon after birth. These includes eyes that slant upward at the outer corners and a lack of muscle tone.

Dyskinesia. A general term for involuntary movements.

Dystonia. Slow, rhythmic, twisting movements.

Early Intervention. The specialized way of interacting with infants to minimize the effects of conditions that can delay early development.

Epicanthic Fold. A fold of skin of the upper eyelid that tends to cover the inner corner of the eye.

Extension. Limbs or trunk becoming straight or extended. The opposite of flexion.

Flexion. The bending of joints.

Floppy. Having weak posture and loose movements.

Genetic. Inherited.

Gross Motor. Relating to the use of the large muscles of the body, such as those in the legs, arms, and abdomen.

Hatha Yoga. The physical aspect of yoga practice—including postures, breathing techniques, cleansing practices, and relaxation.

Hemiplegic. Paralyzed on one side of the body.

Head Control. The ability to control the movements of the head.

High Tone. A tightness or spasticity of the muscles.

Hyperactivity. A specific nervous-system-based difficulty which makes it hard for a person to control muscle (motor) behavior and results in restlessness, fidgeting, and overactive movements.

Hypertonic. An increased tension or spasticity of the muscles. High tone.

Hyposensitive. Partially insensitive to pain.

Hypotonia. Decreased tension of a muscle. Low tone.

I.Q. (Intelligent Quotient). A measure of cognitive ability based on specifically designed standardized tests.

Learning Disability. A disorder in one or more of the basic psychological process involved in understanding or using language, spoken or written, which may manifest itself in an imperfect ability to listen, think, speak, read, write, spell or do mathematical calculations.

Lordosis. An abnormal forward curvature of the spine in the lumbar region.

Low Tone. Decreased muscle tone.

Lower Extremities. The legs.

Lumbar. Relating to the lower back.

Mainstreaming. The practice of involving children with disabilities in regular school and preschool environments.

Mental retardation. Below normal mental function. Children with mental retardation learn more slowly than other children, but "mental retardation" itself does not indicates a specific level of mental ability. The level of mental function may not be identifiable until a much later age.

Microcephaly. Abnormal smallness of the head, accompanied by mild to severe mental retardation and other developmental delays.

Myofascia. The connective membrane around muscle fibers, fiber bundles, and the muscles themselves. Myofascia also forms ligaments and tendons and gives the body its shape.

Muscle Tone. The amount of tension or resistance to movement in a muscle.

Neurodevelopmental Therapy (NDT). A specialized therapy approach that concentrates on encouraging normal movement patterns and discouraging reflexes, postures, and movements. Used by physical, occupational, and speech therapists.

Neuromotor. Involving both nerves and muscles.

Occupational Therapist (OT). A therapist who specializes in improving the development of fine motor and adaptive skills.

Oral Motor. Relating to the movement of muscles in and around the mouth.

Peristalsis. The normal movements of the intestines, moving the food along the digestive tract.

Phenotype. The environmentally and genetically determined observable appearance of an organism, especially as considered with respect to all possible genetically influenced expressions of one specific character.

Physical Therapist (PT). A therapist who specializes in improving the development of gross motor skills.

Porto Alegre. A coastal city in the southernmost region of Brazil.

Prader Willi Syndrome. An inherited disorder that includes obesity, infertility, decreased muscle tone, and mild mental retardation.

Pranayama. Yogic breathing exercises.

Prone. Lying with the front or face downward.

Reflex. An involuntary movement in response to stimulation such as touch, pressure, or joint movement.

Scoliosis. Abdormal lateral curvature of the spine.

Special Needs. Needs generated by a person's disability.

Speech/language Pathologist. A therapist who works to improve speech and language skills, as well to improve oral motor abilities.

Strabismus. Lack of coordinated eye movement resulting in crossing and/or wandering eyes.

Supine. Lying on the back.

Therapist. A trained professional who works to overcome the effects of illness and/or disabilities.

Upper extremities. The arms.

Visual Accommodation. The automatic adjustment in the focal length of the lens of the eye.

Yoga Sutras of Patanjali. This ancient text offers basic instruction on all aspects of the science of yoga.

Bibliography

Bell, Lorna, Eudora Seyfer, and Loena Belland. *Gentle Yoga for People with Arthritis, Stroke Damage, M. S., or People in Wheelchairs.* Gentle Yoga, 1990.

Dewhurst-Maddock, Olivea. *The Book of Sound Therapy.* New York: Simon & Schuster, 1983.

Geralis, Elaine, ed. *Children with Cerebral Palsy: A Parents' Guide.* Bethesda: Woodbine House, 1991.

Iyengar, B. K. S. *Yoga Cien por Cien.* Barcelona: Editorial Miguel Arimany S. A., 1980.

Kuvalayananda, Swami. *Āsanas.* Lonavala, India: Kaivalydhama, 1982.

Lidell, Lucy. *The Sivananda Companion to Yoga.* New York: Simon & Schuster Inc., 1983.

Monro, Robin. *Yoga for Common Ailments.* Fireside, 1991.

Samskrti and Veda. *Hatha Yoga Manual I.* Honesdale, Pennsylvania: The Himalayan International Institute of Yoga Science and Philosophy, 1977.

Satchidananda, Swami. *Integral Yoga Hatha.* Buckingham, VA: Integral Yoga Publications, 1995.

——. *The Yoga Sutras of Patanjali.* Buckingham, VA: Integral Yoga Publications, 1990.

Selikowitz, Mark. *Down Syndrome: The Facts.* Oxford University Press, 1990.

Sivananda, Swami. *A Ciência do Pranayama.* São Paulo: Editora Pensamento, 1993.

Smith, Sally L. *No Easy Answers: The Learning Disabled Child at Home and at School.* New York: Bantam, 1995.

Stray-Gundersen, Karen. *Babies with Down Syndrome: A New Parents Guide.* Bethesda: Woodbine House, 1987.

Stray-Gundersen, Karen, ed. *Babies with Down Syndrome (The Special Needs Collection).* Bethesda: Woodbine House, 1995.

Sumar, Sivakami Sonia. *Yoga para a Criança Especial.* São Paulo: Ground, 1994.

Sumar, Sonia. *Yoga para Excepcionais.* São Paulo: Global/Ground, 1983.

Index

circulation: improving, 95, 126, 132, 179. *See also* heart

Cleansing Breath, 6, 177–178, 227; benefits, 35

cleansing practices, 56

Cobra Pose, 7, 112–113, 144–145, 194–196, 227: advanced variation, 113, 195, 196

colic, 74, 99, 116, 130, 139, 150, 190, 200

colostomy: cautions, 75, 77, 100, 101, 104, 106, 131, 140, 142

concentration: developing, 158, 181, 202; breathing practices for, 179; using stories to develop, 229

constipation, 5, 56, 74, 99, 112, 130, 132, 143, 144, 153, 185, 194

Deep Relaxation, 57, 88–89, 121–122, 168–169, 220–221, 227

demonstrating yoga poses, 173-174

development: how to evaluate your child's, 63-64. *See also* Early Stages of Development

development rates: of different children, 59; of groups of children, 60-61

developmental age, 59

developmental milestones: with yoga control group, 60–62

Devi, Indra, 232

diaphragmatic breathing: benefits, 35

discouragement: facing, 16

disk compression, 78, 107, 116, 150, 152, 183, 200

dorsal-lateral muscles: toning, 203

Down Syndrome: how yoga benefits children with, 54; characteristic features, 4, 28; evaluating a child with, 64; prejudice and, 11, 17. *See also* letters from parents

drawings: use in yoga class, 229

Dynamic Relaxation, 228–229

Early Stage of Development: outline of stages, 59-60

Easy Pose, 8

encouragement, 6, 7, 16, 66, 174. *See also* positive attitude

endocrine glands, 5, 31, 85, 118, 162, 164, 166, 214, 216, 217

energizing: through breath, 179

equilibrium: developing, 30

equipment for yoga, viii

evaluation: of abilities, 5; of motor skills, 63-64; questionnaire for, 61, 67-68

Eye Exercises, 174, 180–182: and strabismus, 10, 12

eye-hand coordination: developing, 181, 182

Fish Pose, 164–165, 216, 227

flexibility: promoted by Sun Salutation, 206

floppy baby syndrome, 4

Focusing, 182

Foot Rotation, 72, 97, 128

To share your comments on this book, to order additional copies, or to request information on Yoga for the Special Child™ Training Programs and Workshops, please contact:

Yoga for the Special Child
Route 1, Box 1559
Buckingham, VA 23921

Telephone: (804) 969-2668
Fax: (804) 969-1962
E-mail: info@specialyoga.com
Website: www.specialyoga.com